Jutta Wohlrab

Happy Birthing Days

A midwife's secret to a joyful, safe and happy birth

RETHINK PRESS

First published in Great Britain 2016
by Rethink Press (www.rethinkpress.com)

Cover image and illustrations © Elin Doka

Contents

A short story

There was once a queen with two gardeners. Each of them planted a precious seed in the ground.

One gardener was very anxious: every day he dug up the seed just to see how it was doing, then planted it again, always worrying about how it would grow and whether it would be all right.

The other gardener would come back to the place where he had planted the seed and sit there, sometimes singing to the seed and talking to it, watering it now and then, and waiting patiently for it to grow. In time he saw the little leaves gently pushing through the soil towards the light...

Which gardener are you?

Introduction

150 babies born every minute!

You can deliver pizza and parcels, but babies should really be **born**!

My name is Jutta and I am a midwife, coach, trainer, international speaker, and the founder of Elements of Birth a. I specialize in supporting women, their partners, and even other birth professionals to achieve a fearless, safe and joyful birth.

I've been a midwife for over thirty years and I've attended over 2,500 births on two continents in every setting from home births to acute hospital care. Thousands more women have been under my care during their pregnancies. This has given me a deep insight into how birth really works, and in combining my solid medical knowledge with complementary therapies, I can offer exceptional solutions to the most common problems.

What is the biggest problem that my mums-to-be face? Mostly, they are either totally confused or very fearful about the upcoming birth, to the point of calling for a Caesarean section (C-section) as they think they will just not be able to handle a normal birth. Even where women are not asking for them, hospitals may just perform them, intervening at a higher rate than ever before. No wonder we are facing a global crisis in birthing, with C-section rates as high as 80 per cent in some countries, according to the Cochrane study.

Add to this a rising rate of maternal mortality and postnatal depression, and the threat to unborn babies from drugs linked to obesity, allergies and asthma, and you have a rather grim picture of what should be the happiest moment in our lives.

This is why I have come up with Happy Birthing Day, the child-birth education system I've taught successfully to hundreds of parents over the last few years. It draws on best practice in a number of disciplines, and gives women confidence and control over their own bodies. It prepares partners to know how to support the mother and to feel part of the whole experience. It's the only course to get people really excited and optimistic about the upcoming birth.

My vision is that women in every corner of the earth should have access to the information that will help them to get the birth they want. Birth is the start of life, and everyone deserves the best start in life.

The idea of writing a book came about at a party with family and friends in the spring of 2013, so thank you to everybody – especially to all the babies around me who seem to have persuaded their mothers to insist that I write a book!

Midwifery may have changed a lot since I became a professional midwife in 1986, but the essence of birth remains the same. The deeper meaning of birth; the fears, doubts, joys that mothers, couples and even midwives sometimes experience – none of this has changed.

At a time when there is so much information about, yet so little understanding of, this amazing process, I feel I must share the learning from thirty years of continuous practice in a range of settings, from home births to birthing centres, primary hospitals and large tertiary hospitals. Working with women in ante- and post-natal care for the last twenty years has also enabled me to develop an extensive understanding of, and expertise in, birthing. Supporting around 2.500 births in three different countries has been the best possible 'school' for me.

At a time when the rate of Caesarean sections remains stubbornly high, showing no signs of diminishing, I feel I must offer all women and their partners the chance to learn about birth, to understand the process and to choose what is best for them. My vision for birth is that every woman should get the fearless, safe and joyful birth she wants.

Birth as part of our life-cycle

Imagine you are a young woman living in a tribe somewhere far from here, in the Amazon perhaps. This is where you grew up and where you have lived all your life. You are part of your tribal community and since you were a small child you have witnessed women and other creatures around you give birth. For you and your sisters, all things in life happen in a natural rhythm. You don't question the rising of the sun in the morning, and the setting of the sun at night. And women giving birth, babies growing up, meeting a partner, making love, and more babies being born are all part of this natural cycle. So are you.

Many of your friends are pregnant, some of them will already have given birth and some are due soon. In your tradition you will already have spent many days together in a secret place, menstruating and learning about what it means to be a woman, but also celebrating, massaging one another, resting, chatting, dancing and singing together.

As a woman, you may have helped your sister give birth, perhaps making a fire, holding her hand, massaging her back, washing her and cooling her down while you whisper soft words of love and support in her ear – you may even have done a little birth dance with her.

You will have seen mums caring for their newborn, breastfeeding them, carrying them and looking after them in a world where it is natural for them just to pick babies up whenever they want to feed, or if they want to poo, or to settle down to sleep with them.

So you would have given birth to your baby in a circle of loving sisters, aunties, mums – many women with birthing skills. Hearing the voices of your sisters, you would have felt the connection to your body and your baby, and trusted your body to bring your sweet baby into the world, just as you have witnessed many times before. You and your baby would have experienced their love and supporting hands from the beginning, and would have had no doubt that you in your turn could be like them. In those cultures the mother is viewed almost like a goddess, since it is she who ensures the natural cycle continues.

 'The wisdom and compassion a woman can intuitively experience in childbirth can make her a source of healing and understanding for other women.'

Stephen Gaskin

But you would also know that nothing is achieved without effort. In your daily life you may have to walk some distance to gather food or water, and collect firewood. You understand that some things just require time and patience to accomplish: when you sow a small seed in the ground, you must wait until a seedling appears, then for that seedling to grow into a big plant.

You are now on the most exciting journey of your life. It is time to move into the flow of life, and to understand at a deep level that you must trust your instincts and let your body take over, using the wisdom and knowledge it has stored since the very beginning of humanity.

My own birth

On a hot Wednesday in May 1963, my mother had been in pre-labour on and off for quite a few days. She had only recently moved to a small town in the south of Germany and my father had to go away for the day for army training. My brother and sister had been taken to my grandmother's place a few hundred kilometres away.

When her labour started in earnest my mother had to ask a neighbour to go and ring my father and ask him to come home. In those days most people did not have a phone at home, so the neighbour had to go to the nearest shop to get in touch with my father.

As soon as he came home, my mother's labour intensified. Having already had two children, my mother knew that the birth was just around the corner. My father wasted no time in driving her to the clinic, and the midwife, who had been in church, was urged to come quickly or the baby would be born without her. Soon after she arrived, I slipped into the world easily, to the great delight of my mother and everyone else in the room. I was then taken away, cleaned, wrapped up and brought back to her, as was the custom in those days.

Later my mother told me that as she held me in her arms, she felt she was holding a very special child, who was looking at the world with wide eyes and wanting to understand everything around her. It is as if through her joyful birth, my mother had given birth to a midwife, so I want to give my deep thanks to my mother and to all mothers. Everyone, no matter what their circumstances, has a mother!

Pregnancy and birth are universal experiences, and I can picture a chain of women from the first one to all the women giving birth today holding hands across the ages. In my memory I also see all the women I have ever cared for and birthed with, holding hands like sisters on a journey.

How to use this book

I have written this book for you and your birthing partners and life partners, to give you an insight into how to prepare for the upcoming birth. I truly believe that the right information and support, together with knowing how to use both your body and your mind, are a winning combination for a great birthing experience, no matter whether you're going to be giving birth at home or in a birth centre or hospital.

In the theory section, I'll give you some inside information about how birth really works, setting the scene for you with useful detail to help you understand this unique process.

In the middle part of the book I'll go into the practicalities of birth. This is the section with 'hands on' exercises: how to breathe, the power of the right touch, making the right sounds, how to move to help your pelvis, and lots more.

In the last part of the book I want to share my experience of how to set the mind in the right direction. There I'll invite you to learn how to set your focus and to let go of unwanted fears and worries, creating positive pictures in your mind.

In fact, the book is like a summary of the childbirth classes that I have been teaching for many years and still teach today. How to get the best out of it? Well, you could just read straight through it, and start doing the daily exercises, or you could go to the sections that are especially relevant to you and read around them. Each chapter can also be read on its own, and will give you some helpful tricks and tips.

Pregnancy, birth – and, of course, what comes after – are part of an amazing journey, so let's get started!

Chapter 1: Birthing theory

Birth: a modern Hollywood drama?

A woman lying on a stretcher, screaming her head off. A siren howls, then an emergency team swarms round her as she huffs and puffs. The baby is born into the medical throng, delivered by smiling hot-shot filmstar obstetrician... The modern picture of birth can be truly scary (but drama sells).

Now forget the Hollywood image, and imagine instead a calm and peaceful atmosphere, quiet, with soft lighting, as a woman gives birth in the water. She will be the one doing the smiling!

Giving birth is a rite of passage, and yet it seems that most women place more faith in their mobile phones and their cars to function efficiently than they do in their own bodies to be able to undertake the process of giving birth successfully. When I speak to women about birth, they reveal their mixed emotions about the process.

But over the years I've also come across many women who, right from the word go, have felt confident and joyful about the forth-coming birth — even some who have said, right after the birth, 'Wow, what was all the fuss about? I could do that again, straight away!'

Like Susanna, thirty-years-old and pregnant with her first baby. When I asked her how she was feeling about the birth, and what preparations she had made, she smiled and said, 'Well, I went to a class with my husband, but that was mainly for his sake. I'm feeling really positive and excited about my pregnancy and the birth. I'm one of four children, and all my life my mother has told me how wonderful it is to be pregnant, and how amazing it is to give birth. So I'm not anxious; I'm looking forward to it.'

A few weeks later I had a call from Susanna. She'd woken up in the night with some contractions and decided after a couple of hours that she should get to the hospital. She woke her husband, he took her there, and a couple of hours after that the baby arrived. Afterwards she thought, 'That was amazing! Was that really all there was to it?' It will come as no surprise to learn that she is now the mother of two beautiful children.

Giving birth is part of a natural rhythm: you grow up, leave childhood, find someone you love and create a baby. Babies are born in different settings — hospitals, birth centres, at home – and into different circumstances. The event of giving birth is itself unique in every case, and could almost be described as a woman. But is she loud and assertive, or gentle and soft? Let her decide on the day.

Come with me now on a journey through all the stages of labour and birth.

What really makes birth happen? An orchestra playing

A woman's body is truly amazing. Throughout her pregnancy different hormones, working in harmony, will be supporting the whole process, making sure that the baby is growing well and that the mother's body is getting ready for the birth. In fact, I picture an orchestra playing.

Birth is like a beautiful piece of music. Imagine you are going to a concert. You relax, have a chat, and maybe something to eat while the orchestra is tuning up, then you find your seat. This is the pre-labour period, as the musicians — the birth hormones — arrive and prepare to start playing in harmony. Once they are all present and correct, and in tune, the music — the process of birth — begins. What you don't know, of course, is what sort of music it will be: will it be calm and reflective, focused inwards, or will it be wild and demonstrative, expressing emotions freely? This is something you will find out for yourself when your time comes.

From around thirty-seven weeks you may experience some small contractions and some tingly sensations. Some of these are to position the baby well in the uterus, and some are to prepare your body for the birth. These are signs that the hormones that come into play in the process of childbirth are starting to act. From this point on birth could happen at any time.

Progesterone

Progesterone, one of the female hormones that belongs to the steroids group, actually helps women to become pregnant. Once the egg has become embedded in the uterus, the placenta takes over the production of progesterone, which also helps to produce oestrogen and testosterone.

So what does progesterone actually do? In early pregnancy it helps the lower part of the abdomen to relax, so that the pregnancy can grow and thrive. During your pregnancy your cervix is about three to four centimetres long: this makes sure that the baby is well protected in the womb. Progesterone will help to shorten and soften your cervix, and open it up. The cervix can shorten and soften over a period of many weeks or in just a few days. Some women have described a stinging or a tingly sensation in their vagina, which can be a sign that the uterus is getting ready. Other women don't feel anything at all.

Like relaxin, progesterone helps the pelvis to open up to accommodate the birth.

Progesterone itself produces oestrogen, and progesterone and oestrogen are like two sisters working together throughout pregnancy and childbirth. In fact, is there anything progesterone does not do? It must be the first violin of the hormone orchestra.

Prostaglandin

Prostaglandin is another key player in the hormone orchestra, vital to enable the body to release the baby, and connecting and reacting to all the other hormones in a finely tuned balance.

Sperm contains a natural prostaglandin, which raises the question of whether it's safe to make love during your pregnancy. The good news is yes, if you have a normal pregnancy. In the last weeks of pregnancy your cervix starts to get shorter and softer (see above). There are also receptors inside the cervix that ripen at the end of pregnancy, and this is where your partner can help in a very natural way. Of course, you can make love all the way through pregnancy, but towards the end the prostaglandins in the sperm will help the cervix to soften and prepare for the birth. He helped the baby in, so he can help him/her out!

Research has shown that women who had regular sex from the thirty-sixth week of pregnancy needed fewer interventions during the birth itself — no doubt because of extra production of these clever hormones.

Oxytocin (the love hormone!)

Once oxytocin arrives, labour can start.

Oxytocin is an amazing agent and has been widely researched in recent years — whole books have been written about it. Both men and women produce oxytocin, though women seem to have a higher level of it. Oxytocin belongs to the category of sexual hormones that enable a certain group of muscles to contract in a wave-like motion. During sex it helps us to reach orgasm, and it also supports the process of birth. It even provides some natural pain relief during birth, takes away fear, and helps you to forget any pain after it

Oxytocin is called the love hormone, and plays a key part in bonding. It floods both body and brain. When a couple make love, it is oxytocin that makes them want to melt into each other. But we even produce oxytocin when, for example, we are sitting around having a meal with friends and feeling very connected with them.

It is oxytocin that stimulates the frequent contractions required to give birth, but once the baby is born, oxytocin is also released when a woman looks at her baby for the first time, giving rise to the vital bond she will have with her child. Skin to skin contact at this stage promotes an even stronger connection, and breast-feeding produces a huge flush of oxytocin throughout the body, from the head to the stomach. The gut is in fact our second brain, with large numbers of oxytocin receptors!

The hormone that is such an important part of sexuality is also vital for giving birth — that's only natural!

Tip

Avoid synthetic oxytocin: your brain cannot process it. Natural oxytocin is released in pulses, whereas the artificial stuff will hit you like a rocket and will not give you the feelings of connectedness, happiness or euphoria that natural oxytocin brings.

Adrenalin and its sister catecholamine

A woman's body will produce a lot of other hormones during birth, but these will only be helpful if released at the right moment.

Unfortunately, if your 'fight or flight' mechanism is triggered during birth, other hormones, such as adrenalin and cate-cholamine, take over. In the presence of these hormones, very little oxytocin is produced. If you think you are in danger, the process of birth will stall.

In an experiment conducted many years ago, a pregnant mouse was put into a small cage and started giving birth. After a while a researcher sprayed some cat urine into the cage. Guess what? The mouse stopped giving birth until she was moved into a clean cage, and once she felt safe and secure she continued to give birth.

This little mouse demonstrates very clearly how birth works. Adrenalin and its sister catecholamine are fantastic if you are running for your life, or going for gold, but they are definitely not helpful when you are in the process of opening up for childbirth. If you are releasing a high volume of stress hormones, you will be unable to release the required amount of oxytocin at the same time.

If these stress hormones are produced once labour has progressed quite a long way, it can lead to foetal eject reflex — the baby is born in double quick time, much as if it had used an ejector seat!

Case study: letting go

The following story shows how the progress of birth can change, and, more importantly, can be changed.

In a home birth practice in Berlin in the early nineties I met a woman called Ute. She was already the mother of a lovely little girl who had been discovered at eight months to have a genetic disorder. She needed a lot of extra support and care, but was much loved by both her parents.

When Ute became pregnant for the second time, she went for a genetic check-up and had some extra tests done to see if her new baby would be healthy. Once all the checks had shown there was nothing to fear, Ute was very relieved and booked in to the birth centre where I was working. I met Ute and her husband many times during her pregnancy and we established a good relationship.

Ute's due date came and went, and we continued to meet for regular check-ups. At ten days overdue, I asked her how she was feeling and reassured her that it wouldn't be long before the baby was born. One night I had a dream that Ute gave birth, and when I saw her for a check-up the following day, she told me that the assistants at her daughter's kindergarten had also dreamt that the new baby had been born.

A day later Ute rang me in the morning and told me that she had had fairly strong contractions. I was excited, too, and asked her to come in. Once she arrived it was clear labour was well established, and everything then progressed very quickly. But when Ute finally had the urge to push, she started holding back, crying, and shouting 'No, no, no!' I sensed that she was afraid that something might be wrong with her new baby — I could feel her anxiety and doubts rolling over her and towards me like a rushing wave.

So I asked her to take a breath and release it, and said to her: 'Now is the time to say yes. Whatever will be will be, and you must understand this. Whatever the baby is like, you must let it out, so please let it go, and say 'Yes''. It took a couple more minutes, and a bit more reassurance till Ute finally yelled 'Yes, baby, yessss' and a beautiful little boy emerged into the world. He was perfect, and he was welcomed with a lot of relief, tears, and strong surges of emotion. When his special sister was brought from her kindergarten to meet him an hour later, she fell in love with him straight away.

Women and their individual stories amaze me in my work every day.

Prolactin: the mothering hormone

As with oxytocin, prolactin is a hormone that directs the mother's love even as it prepares her for breastfeeding. During pregnancy prolactin will have increased the density of the milk ducts. Stimulated by endorphins and oxytocin during the birth, prolactin enables to brain to reorganise its focus after the birth.

All three hormones are produced deep in the primal part of our brain, and this is just one of the reasons why women in labour should be left undisturbed as far as possible. The ears and eyes are gateways into the brain, so it's best to avoid any stimuli that interfere with the deep flow of labour, and the well-tuned process orchestrated by the magical cocktail of hormones.

Right after the birth, the mother will look at her baby, and the baby will look back at her: the oxytocin will be flowing, but prolactin will also be promoting her focus on, and pleasure in, the baby, helping her to become a mother. As the adrenalin produced at the end of labour recedes, the mother will want to settle back, cuddle her baby and start breastfeeding. The little baby itself will actually start to search for the breast. Prolactin and oxytocin will take over from adrenalin, helping the colostrum, the very first milk, to flow and stimulating the delivery of the placenta.

Prolactin is amazing in that it not only produces breast milk, it also contains breast milk, and breastfeeding leads to a feeling of warmth and security that both mother and baby enjoy. It also helps babies' brains to develop. What's not to like?

Making the most of mother's little helpers

It's great to go with the oxytocin flow during birth, and for this reason it's very helpful to support women in labour to stay positive.

Playing along with the orchestra of hormones in this beautiful song of labour will be the **endorphins** your body will release. They come in a natural flow, of their own accord, making you feel happy and strong; they give the feeling of being in a trance and get you into the zone. Whenever you hear stories of mothers lifting a car to save their trapped child, you know that it's the endorphins that will have given them the strength. Endorphins allow you to fly high towards your goal, on a roll and losing all awareness of time and space. Endorphins must be invited to the birth party.

To release helpful levels of endorphins, and, consequently, **dopamine**, it's important to feel that you are doing well, and this has special significance during birth. Unfortunately people in general are very good at telling themselves what they can't do.

If you're uncertain about your skills and abilities, it feels really good when someone praises you, and it builds your confidence and your faith in your skills. Remember how you felt at school: however much you had prepared for a test, all it would take was a quizzical look or a doubtful sound from a teacher as they passed to make you think, 'Oh no, this is rubbish. I'd better cross it out and start all over again.' If the teacher had passed by with a positive face and an encouraging murmur, you would have been more likely to feel, 'Yeah, I'm actually doing this and I'm doing it well.'

So give dopamine a chance: it will make you feel as if you're giving yourself a round of applause and that's good. The better supported you are, and the less doubt you feel, the easier it is to give birth to a baby.

I can't emphasise enough that the key to a successful birth is for a woman to feel secure, encouraged and supported.

The physiology of labour

The pre-birthday party and your due date
Birth is an amazing process, and it really is worth the time and effort to understand it, even though every woman's take on it will be individual.

Everything in nature has a rhythm: the sun rises and sets every day, the moon waxes and wanes, the tides ebb and flow. Similarly, the pregnant body prepares itself for birth, and labour starts once a rhythm has been established. Many first-time mothers worry that they won't pick up the signs of labour and will miss the moment when they have to ring the midwife or the hospital.

Although they might be very fearful about the forthcoming birth, some simultaneously harbour a concern that they might miss it, and end up having given birth without knowing that it's going to happen.

I can't help but smile at these contradictory feelings, but in fact it's quite understandable: most people today have little knowledge of the process of birth. We no longer live in large families and only a very small number of babies are born at home, so few women have a chance to witness a baby being born before they give birth to their own child.

So how can you know when you are likely to go into labour? First of all, normal labour can start any time between thirty-seven and forty-two weeks of gestation. Any time during those weeks is considered normal. In fact, only about 2 to 4% of babies are actually born on their due date, and if you are smart you will give your family and friends a due date two weeks after the real one. Nothing is worse than well-meaning friends constantly calling you around the time of the due date to ask you if you've had your baby yet! If they don't hear from you, they are likely to disturb your well-earned nap, saying they were sure you must have had it by now, which doesn't make you feel any better if you are over your due date.

The best laid plans
Although birth somehow always comes as a surprise, many women tap into their intuition and might have dreams, feelings and visions about the birth to come. But when woman plans, the goddess laughs, as the saying goes.

Case study: late baby

I planned a birth with a friend of mine who was expecting her second baby. She is a very intuitive person and was convinced that her baby would be born before the due date. We agreed that the birth should take place either at a birthing centre or at her home, depending on where I was going to be when the day arrived.

Everything was ready at her home, including plans for her first child to be looked after. We were both busy with major events, and the due date came and went with no baby in sight. More days passed.

A famous swami came to visit, and we both went and got blessings from her. Even she told us that the birth was just around the corner. My friend was now close to being ten days overdue, and we had started to have the 'what if' conversation.

I went to see her on the morning that she was ten days overdue. We had a chat and I gave her a lovely treatment: hypnosis, deep relaxation with visualisation of letting go of things, and some acupuncture to stimulate her body. I left her at lunchtime, assuring her that it could be only couple of hours, or at most a couple of days, before the baby arrived. Her husband rang a few hours later to ask me if she should go into the birthing pool. I decided to go round there, even though my friend had told me that nothing was likely to happen for a few hours. When I got there I found that labour was in full swing, and two hours later she gave birth to a beautiful baby boy.

I'm telling you this story to show that even though you may have a compelling intuition and a strong connection to your body, sometimes labour just hides and does her own thing — and that's fine. One thing is for sure: every baby will be born, just as the sun rises every day. As with most things in life, it requires love, trust and patience: some things just take time.

The stages of labour and why you should make a chocolate cake

If you were planning to climb Mount Everest you'd probably take a look at the map to see where you were actually going. As giving birth is also an important undertaking, you'll probably want to understand a bit about the process and the different stages it goes through.

Birth is an amazing journey, and some women travel on an express train while others take their time. Let's find out what's going to happen.

Normal labour can start at any time between thirty-seven and forty-two weeks. At a certain stage the receptors in your cervix are going to get ready, and will be more likely to respond to the hormonal call of your body. We are still not quite sure who or what it is that actually triggers the birth: is it the baby? Is it the mother? Or is it something in the placenta? The jury is still out. What is certain is that once the baby and your body are both ready, birth will be just around the corner.

Labour is traditionally described as having three stages, and yet there is a fourth one: pre-labour. Pre-labour has its own highly significant place and purpose in the process.

Pre-labour

Imagine pre-labour as your body running through a last-minute checklist to make sure that everything is in order for the birth. Your womb, the expert in these matters, is going to do some warming-up exercises. This means that in the days before the actual birth your uterus will start to contract and then stop again. These contractions might go on for some hours, making you think your time has come..., and then they'll stop again. This can be quite nerve-wracking, so it's important to understand what is going on.

Before thirty-seven weeks the baby floats freely above the pelvic rim. (If you are expecting your second or third, or a subsequent baby, you may find that the baby will spend a little longer floating above the pelvic rim and will only engage once labour starts.) At around thirty-seven weeks the head becomes engaged in the pelvis in a process called lightening. You might already have felt a bit of pulling and stretching. These light contractions are designed to get the baby in touch with the pelvis and move its head deeper into the pelvis, that is, to engage. But this process does not lead directly to labour, and it may be followed by a few weeks in which you will only experience the odd contraction now and then.

You can help your baby get into a good position during your pregnancy by moving your pelvis in a certain way, and by spending more time on all fours. Chapter 8 will give you more information about this.

Tip

If everything is going well, stay at home for as long as possible. Your hormones will be flowing well, and it's less likely they will be disturbed.

Once this 'settling' process has taken place, you might find that towards evening you begin to feel mild to medium, or even fairly strong, contractions that will be very uncoordinated, sometimes coming quickly one after the other, and sometimes with big pauses in between.

BUT in nature everything has a rhythm the sun rises and sets, the seasons come and go and so does birth. As long as your contractions lack rhythm, the birth will be soon, but labour won't have started yet.

At this stage the most important thing is to relax, relax, and relax some more. This is not the time to try to 'bring it on' or make the contractions stronger. It's the time to take it easy, and it's a great time to give your birth breathing a trial run. The contractions might continue on into labour, or they might stop after a couple of hours.

 'Muscles send messages to each other. Clenched fists, a tight mouth, a furrowed brow, all send signals to the birth-passage muscles, the very ones that need to be loosened. Opening up to relax these upper-body parts relaxes the lower ones.'

William and Martha Sears

So what's the best thing to do? I promise you that you won't miss out on your own birth, so welcome this opportunity to limber up for the big event, but to make yourself comfortable as well. Now is the time to eat, drink and watch a funny film. You should have lots of funny films around at home in the run-up to the birth as it's very helpful if you're already in the pre-labour stage to have a good laugh and release some happy hormones. This is a great way to make you, your body and your baby feel really good.

Watching a film might not be every woman's cup of tea, but in my experience what is helpful is to focus on something else, especially at the beginning. Remember that this might just be a trial warm-up, and not yet the real deal. Making yourself comfortable on your sofa with a hot water bottle or taking a bath can be just as good for taking your mind off things or you could even bake a big chocolate cake.

Case study: timing

Take Gabrielle. Gabrielle was expecting her first baby, and she rang me, unsure about whether she should be heading for the hospital. From what she told me, it sounded to me as if she was in the pre-labour phase: some of the contractions were stronger than others, and also she was clearly able to chat to me quite effortlessly. I reassured her that this was just a trial run and that she should stay at home for the time being.

Now this went on for a few days. Gabrielle would have some contractions, but after a couple of hours they would stop, and she would wake up still pregnant. One day when she was having sporadic contractions, Gabrielle decided to bake a chocolate cake to take her mind off things. What a great idea that was! By the time the cake was ready labour was well established, so Gabrielle, her partner and the chocolate cake went off to give birth. We all enjoyed a large and well-deserved slice of it straight after her baby was born.

Some women will tell you that they spent days and days in labour, and I suspect that in fact they spent much of this time in pre-labour. It could be that their baby was not well-positioned in the pelvis, and that their uterus was trying very hard to correct this. In this case, it can be helpful to move your pelvis, and to ask a midwife or someone at your birthing centre to feel for how the baby is located, and if need be to do some pelvic movements to correct the position.

Don't forget that this phase is not going to last forever. Taking warm baths and showers, taking as many naps as you can between surges — these are all great ways to conserve your energy.

And if you do find that your pre-labour is very intense, goes on for several days and causes great discomfort, you should consult a professional who can check on the baby's position and help you to move it into a good position. One woman whom I had been helping with hypnosis rang me, although she was in the care of another midwife, because she had been in great discomfort for some days. I explained to her how she needed to move her hips to swing the baby towards the front, and how to lie down. This helped her labour to start and the birth went really well.

And while some women will experience pre-labour, others will just go straight into the first stage of labour.

Signs that labour has arrived

How will you know that labour has started, and that you should contact the hospital, birthing place or your midwife?

The mucus plug

The first thing to happen could be that you lose your mucus plug. If the discharge is sticky, it is the mucus plug that was situated in your cervix, acting as a barrier protecting the baby. It could be clear, or it could have some tiny bits of brownish-coloured blood in it. If it contains a bit more blood, it is called a bloody show. Sometimes the plug comes out because you have been examined, or because you have made love, and sometimes just for no reason.

Some women become very 'juicy' at the end of their pregnancy, and do not lose their mucus plug all in one go.

Losing the mucus plug is not counted as a secure sign that the birth is close, so there is no need to contact anyone at this stage.

The amniotic fluid

What, then, is the real sign of being in labour? If you begin to lose amniotic fluid, which is called the release (or rupture) of the amniotic membrane, you may experience a constant trickle of fluid, showing that there is a small leakage. Or you may experience a flood of liquid, or wake up to find you are lying in a puddle of fluid. I can assure you you haven't peed in your pants.

What you need to do now is check the colour of the fluid: as long as it is clear, pink, or very light-yellowish, you're fine. It's time to change your undies, observe that your baby is moving, and get in touch with your place of care – different rules apply in different countries, but wherever you are you will need to let your practitioner know what is happening.

If when you check, you see a bright green fluid, or a browner one that looks like pea soup, you need to get in touch with your practitioner without delay. This will mean that your baby has done a poo in the fluid, and it should be monitored for its own safety.

Tip
Kiss, dance, massage and celebrate the start of your birthing journey with your partner.

How long?

One in four women will start to release their fluid prematurely, and it can take some time – days, even – before labour really starts. In Germany you will have a maximum of twenty-four hours after the release of fluid, whereas in Australia you might be allowed to go for as long as five days, under daily observation, before it is acknowledged that the process of birth has begun. Different countries take different approaches.

Case study: membrane rupture

My lovely friend, let's call her Susanna, was pregnant with her first child and planned to give birth in a birthing centre. Her membrane ruptured, the fluid was clear, the baby was fine, and there was no infection. Every day she came in to the birthing centre for a check-up. On Day Two she began having acupuncture sessions.

She was getting a little nervous about when labour would actually start, as she really didn't want an induction. But finally, on Day Five, she woke up with mild contractions, which she was happy to manage by herself. When they got stronger she woke her husband. They lit some candles, played some music, danced and kissed for a while. They rang me at about 7.00 a.m., on the way to the birthing centre.

When I got there at around 8.00, labour was well established. Susanna spent some time in the bath, walked for a while, rested on all fours, and her beautiful baby girl was finally born on the birthing stool at around lunchtime. The five-day wait had certainly been worthwhile.

I've passed this story on to you because it certainly taught me a lot about different approaches to birth. It's worth having a chat to the professionals where you live to understand how they do things, and to buy some extra time for yourself if it's needed.

Contractions

The strength and frequency of contractions are another indication of how well established labour is. If you have been having contractions every three to five minutes over a period of two hours, and you find you cannot chat while having one, labour is definitely well under way, and you should call your midwife or go to wherever you are booked in for your delivery. If you are expecting your second or third child, you will need to react faster than with a first baby. But bear in mind that these are just estimates, and you should listen to your instincts.

If you arrive at the hospital or birthing centre with labour in full swing, you will of course stay and give birth. If it turns out to be a false alarm, don't worry. If you are given the option of going home, you should definitely do so. Home is the best place to be: it's familiar, you can relax there and you will feel more comfortable.

Finally...

Don't forget that even once you are fully dilated, it could still be hours until your baby is born and placed in your arms. Even if things speed up, I know from experience that you will be able to feel that this is happening. Trust in the sensations you are experiencing and allow yourself to check in with your body to understand what's good and what works for you. And consult the midwife: most of the time she will be able to assess how far advanced your labour is by talking to you. There is nothing more exciting!

Pay attention: when to contact your midwife or doctor

So far, of course, I've been describing what happens during a 'normal' pregnancy. Now I need to tell you about signs to be alert to – signs that should ring alarm bells:

✳ From about the seventeenth to the twenty-second week of your pregnancy, depending on whether it is your first or a subsequent baby, you should start to feel movement: a little, light fluttery movement like butterfly wings touching you. (At the beginning women sometimes think it is just a bit of wind, but you will notice the rhythmical tap, tap, tapping.) Once this is established you should feel a minimum of ten movements in twenty-four hours. The more advanced you are in your pregnancy, the more clearly you should feel this minimum of ten movements a day. If you feel very little movement or none at all, you should have a big drink of iced water and eat something sugary. You should get some major movement in about thirty minutes, but if not, go and get your baby checked out.

✳ If you get strong bleeding, go straight to hospital, as there could be a problem with your placenta.

✳ If at any time you feel really unwell, or suffer from blurred vision and a bad headache, get in touch with your practitioner.

It's important to understand what is normal and what needs further investigation. Please trust your intuition, and consult the medical practitioner who is looking after you, asking questions whenever you are unsure. And don't forget that pregnancy and childbirth are natural procedures that in most cases go smoothly.

The first stage: opening up

As I explained in the section on hormones, once prostaglandin has done its job and the cervix is soft and already a little bit open, oxytocin will be released to get the uterus moving in a wave-like motion. At the same time, the baby begins to push a little with its feet, so that uterus and baby are working together as a team.

In the first stage of labour the contractions will become more rhythmical, and they will move the baby down onto the cervix — the neck of the womb — which will help the cervix to open up gently. How does that work? First of all, the hormones that women produce throughout their pregnancy make the pelvis become softer and able to open up like a flower. Relaxin enables the pelvis to become 2.5 to 3.5 centimetres wider than it was before pregnancy. Isn't it amazing how so many different processes combine to allow for the birth of a child!

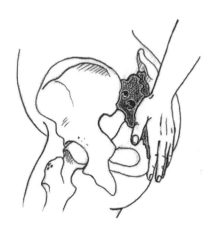

The pelvis opens up like a flower

What is a contraction? A contraction is a wave-like motion of the uterus that usually lasts around forty-five to sixty seconds. You will usually be unable to speak while you are having one. This is nature's way of focusing our minds more on ourselves and the process of birth, of making sure we're not too busy chatting, phoning, emailing or doing something else to stop and deliver a baby.

In the first stage of labour the baby is moving down into the birth canal to push gently on the cervix with its head. This movement onto the cervix sends a message to the brain, which releases more oxytocin. This in itself is not enough for the baby to be born, because birth is in fact teamwork. During the process of birth, the baby will make itself as small as possible, tucking its chin into its chest and moving through the pelvis in a spiral motion with the minimum of resistance, like a button gliding through a buttonhole. This process could take three hours or it could thirteen or more.

Of course women cannot feel by how many centimetres their cervix is already open, but many report feeling that the baby is shifting further down.

Case study: stuck in labour

In a small hospital in Berlin, I looked after one woman in labour whose waters had broken and whose cervix was about four to five centimetres dilated. Unfortunately the hospital setting and the pressure Betty felt put her labour on hold. She was stuck in the middle of her labour, but she did not want to be induced. We tried many different things, such as acupuncture and homeopathy, but for some reason none of these did the trick. The pressure from the doctors to move the labour on was growing, so I suggested that Betty and her partner kiss and hug, and try some nipple stimulation. Since the hormones associated with giving birth and with making love are the same, this technique can work well.

I left the birthing room to give the couple some space, and sure enough I was called in thirty minutes later to find that the contractions had picked up beautifully. I advised them to keep up the good work... After another thirty minutes I was called in again, and Betty told me that with the contractions she had clearly felt the baby moving down. To my delight a healthy and beautiful baby was born just an hour later.

Some women are very much in tune with their bodies and can feel these fine differences, while others may be so overwhelmed by the experience of labour that they don't distinguish sensations in this way. Either way is cool. You may not know whether you're three or seven centimetres dilated, but you will know how you feel.

The first stage of labour is complete once your cervix is fully open, to an estimated ten centimetres.

The second stage of labour

Often the birthing body will take a little break before it progresses on to the next stage of birth — what an amazing process! And what's more, your baby is going to help; it will make itself as small as possible, turning and gently pushing itself down with its feet. I'm very sure babies want to be born and want to help their mothers. After all, this is a team effort.

From the moment your cervix is fully dilated it could take from thirty minutes to three hours for the baby to show itself. This is a fluid period of labour, with much depending on the circumstances. Birth does not have a built-in clock; you must rely on the signs that will tell you and those around you that things are changing.

One very obvious sign could be that you have an urge to go to the toilet. A lot of women feel as if they are going to have a bowel movement, and I am usually delighted when a woman tells me she wants to use the toilet. Apart from anything else, the toilet is a great place for privacy and for feeling you can let yourself go, and in a hospital setting it is often the only place where you can remain undisturbed. Being in a calm and supportive atmosphere is absolutely vital.

Once the baby starts shifting down towards the pelvic floor, the game often starts to change. You might feel a mild, or even a really strong urge to push. What is happening is that the pressure of the baby's head on the pelvic floor is triggering the feeling of wanting to push, and this will activate certain hormones again. Picture the baby sitting on a slide and needing to get itself round a bend. The midwife can often see a the baby's head deep inside, showing itself little by little as the uterus pushes the baby down and out.

Tip
Picture a slide, with the baby sliding down it and out into the world.

The baby may be coming down the slide quickly, or it may be coming down slowly. Often a woman may feel that nothing is happening at all, which makes her quite desperate. It's quite typical at this stage for women to become very emotional, maybe even declaring that they cannot do it. Some may even vomit, cry out for help, while others remain very focused. However, a woman approaches it, this is the final step — the step that will transform women into mothers and men into fathers.

With each gentle push, with each moan and pant and groan, the baby moves down, stretching the muscles of the vagina. The vagina in its turn, with a wave-like motion, massages the baby further down and out. There comes a point where the baby's head moves up a little and back again. Women might not feel this happening, or they might feel a burning or a stinging sensation as the baby's head starts to emerge – to crown. The baby's hairline is positioned under the pubic bones, and both mother and baby use the leverage this provides to move the head up so that it can be born. The head should emerge slowly as the soft tissue of the vagina and the perineum need a little time to stretch open fully and let the baby out. In most cases once the head is born the rest of the body will emerge with the next contraction. A baby is born ready to go into your waiting arms.

The third stage of labour

The moment a baby is born is just beyond words. You could peep into a birthing room and tell that a baby has been born just from the look of bliss on the faces of the people in the room.

The third stage of labour is just as important as all the other stage, and has a deeper significance than we often credit it with; everyone in the delivery room should be aware of this. The birth is really only complete once the placenta has been born and mother and baby are well. But to reach this position the birth process needs to continue undisturbed. Straight after the birth all the senses are alive and open to this crucial stage of connection and survival. The contact between the pair must begin in a warm and secure environment.

Both the mother's and the baby's body will be flooded with high levels of oxytocin after the birth. The stratospheric levels of this amazing cocktail of love and ecstasy are unique to this moment. This makes sure that the two of them can bond really well, but it also helps the placenta to be delivered really easily.

'*It is not only that we want to bring about an easy labour, without risking injury to the mother or the child; we must go further. We must understand that childbirth is fundamentally a spiritual, as well as a physical, achievement. The birth of a child is the ultimate perfection of human love.*'

Dr Grantly Dick-Read, 1953

Skin-to-skin contact, looking into each other's eyes, and the baby nuzzling, licking and feeding from the breast; all these things also help to keep the uterus contracted, preventing haemorrhaging after the birth. The baby can feel, smell and hear, connecting through the warmth of the mother's body and her soft touch.

Another key feature of this stage is the support that the baby continues to receive through the umbilical cord. Inside the womb the baby is well supplied with blood coming from the placenta. In fact the nutrient-rich placenta is brilliant at multi-tasking, fulfilling the roles of the lungs, kidneys, liver and gut for the unborn baby. (See Chapter 5 for a detailed description of how the placenta works.)

After the birth the placenta continues to deliver small amounts of blood to the baby through the umbilical cord with each contraction. This is a cunning plan to get the baby off to the best start in life. Babies get great benefits from late or delayed cord clamping, and recent studies have shown that if this process is allowed to continue as long as there is a pulsing sensation in the placenta, around 100 to 150 millilitres of blood can be transmitted to the baby. Bearing in mind that the total volume of a baby's blood is only around 300 to 350 millilitres, it looks as though the placental blood probably contains the best 'stem cells' you could give your baby. In fact, a recent study shows that babies in need of resuscitation benefit greatly from staying on the cord and being supported by its natural systems.

Even babies that are breathing independently should have the chance to get the support from the cord that they deserve. It seems that they control the amount of blood coming through the cord by their crying: when they cry very little blood comes through the cord, but when they rest a greater volume flows through. Nature's fine tuning of this process is just amazing!

But there comes a time when you must finally get let go of the placenta. It has done its job, and it needs to come out somewhere between thirty minutes and two hours after the birth. Bear in mind, though, that these are estimates, as every hospital or birth centre will have its own practices, and much will depend on how your birth goes and what medication you had. The birth of the placenta will be much easier than the birth of the baby as it is very soft.

Case study: delivering the placenta

What can happen is that after the birth a woman is so relaxed that it can be difficult for her to produce another 'release'. I remember one woman I attended in a birthing centre I was working for at the time. Kathrin had had a straightforward birth, and she and her partner were happily snuggling up with the baby, but the placenta showed no signs of wanting to emerge. Since Kathrin was fine and everything was going well I didn't worry, but when the placenta hadn't shown up after two hours we started to try to get it moving: breastfeeding, going to the toilet, and other things. One of the policies of the birthing centre was that a doctor should be informed if the placenta had not been delivered within two hours of the birth. Luckily the doctor on duty was very busy, and just before Susan was to be sent off to the operating theatre she suddenly had an urge to push and released a beautiful and complete placenta.

Looking back I'd say it was about four hours before the placenta was born, but it was as if Susan was so wrapped up in her baby that, though she could have delivered it sooner, her body did not want the distraction. Most placentas will be born much more quickly!

Once the placenta is out, your midwife will have a feel of your uterus, and will examine the placenta to make sure that it is complete, and that none of it has remained in the uterus.

But it's important not to overlook the significance of the placenta throughout pregnancy and even after the birth – have a look at Chapter 5.

The womb: your expert

Throughout the whole of your pregnancy, just as throughout the whole of your life, the presence and the levels of your hormones are changing continuously. Even now, we don't really understand all the hormones that are at work during pregnancy and birth.

In the last trimester of your pregnancy, the body will start to produce a huge amount of **relaxin**, a hormone to open up and soften your body, giving it more flexibility and allowing the pelvis itself to open up a little more.

At around the same time your **oestrogen** levels are going up, and it is this that I feel gives women the beautiful soft look that makes them so special. All cultures need women to be pregnant and to give birth, so it's no wonder that in so many of them a pregnant woman was treated like a goddess and honoured for her fertility. So honour yourself, and remember that you are beautiful at all stages throughout this amazing process!

Throughout your body there are different receptors that respond to hormonal signals at different times in different ways. There are **prostaglandin** receptors in the cervix, and some women feel a tingly or slightly stinging sensation in their cervix. If a woman is going to give birth for the first time, her cervix feels like the tip of your nose; if a woman has given birth before, her cervix feels more like soft lips that are lightly open. If you are very curious, you can feel this for yourself. To prepare the cervix the cervix for the birth, you can

* make love regularly from thirty-six weeks onwards, since sperm contains a natural prostaglandin; and

* drink two cups of raspberry leaf tea a day, as it, too, contains a natural prostaglandin.

You could also help to prepare your cervix for the birth by having acupuncture once a week from thirty-six weeks. A large study done in Germany showed that women who received stimulation to certain acupuncture points once a week had a better experience at the birth itself, including fewer interventions. I have worked with acupuncture since 1995, and opened the first official acupuncture practice for women inside this hospital, offering it to all the women who came there to give birth. It has made a huge difference and is now widely available in Germany.

The uterus at thirty-seven weeks

At around thirty-seven weeks, your uterus will be quite big, and it may well want to exercise a bit. The irregular contractions that women experience around this time may lead to feelings of insecurity and uncertainty. But these contractions are very important, since they help the baby to move lower and become well-positioned in the pelvis. That way she will be able to find her way down and out more easily. The key to a good birth is to have all the components in order.

'There is no other organ quite like the uterus. If men had such an organ, they would brag about it.'

Ina May Gaskin,
founder of the Farm Midwifery Centre

That the uterus often needs to correct the position of the baby is a result of our modern lifestyle. Women spend a lot time tilting their bodies and their pelvises backwards. Lying on a couch, sitting in a car with a seatbelt on, spending hours in front of a computer — all these postures invite the baby to turn his spine towards the mother's back, whereas the ideal position is for the baby's back to be under her belly. If the spine is more tilted towards the back, of if the baby is not sitting well in the pelvis, the body will try to correct the position of the baby as best it can, leading to those contractions you will experience at thirty-seven weeks: your body is preparing, your body is getting ready.

10 cm: is that all?

In the process of labour your Oxytocin is delivered in pulses which allows the uterus to move in a wave like motion. The cervix is going to pull back, to disappear. You cannot feel the extent of dilation, but you can sometimes feel the process, and how the baby is moving further down.

The cervix opens up to an estimated 10cm across during the time of the birth, and once it has achieved this dimension, it is what the midwife would call 'fully dilated'. No one will be wielding a tape measure: this will be established through an examination, or through other external signs that tell the midwife that you have reached this point in your journey.

In some countries you will be examined more frequently than in others, depending on the culture, although less is more in this respect: examining you every two hours to identify your progress is not going to speed up your labour one bit. Even once you are fully dilated, it could still be another two to three hours until the baby is born.

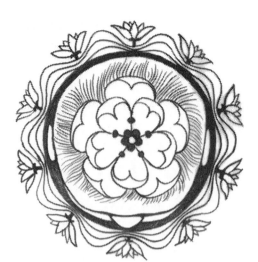

Your visual mandala: can you see the baby's face in it?

Case study: visualising the dilation

One day I was birthing with a women who had taken my birth preparation class. As she was sitting in the bath, I noticed that with every contraction she held up a little saucer with a lovely pattern on it. She had measured it and found it to be 10 cm across, so she held it up to remind herself of the 10 cm the cervix has to dilate to for the baby to be born. You could copy the mandala below to create your own visual aid.

The length of a labour is a highly individual matter, and does not lend itself to measurements, rules and predictions. Imagine you are a gardener looking at a tree laden with fruit. The individual fruits are kind of ready at around the same time, but not simultaneously. Some will need longer than others. It's just the same with pregnancy and childbirth: the length of the process does not diminish the quality of the birth. Forget about time and just go with the flow.

Finally, if you are having a vaginal birth after a C-section or at risk of having to be induced, a study in the UK has shown that it can be useful to have a regular 'strip and stretch' done by a midwife from around thirty-seven weeks, assuming your cervix is already in a favourable condition (that is, softer, shorter, and a little bit open). The midwife will examine you vaginally and gently massage the cervix. There is no risk of it bringing on the birth, it simply gets your cervix ready for the birth.

The placenta and its functions

The placenta plays such a significant part throughout the whole pregnancy and birth that sometimes I feel we should honour it a bit more than we do. From just being a clump of cells that merge and grow, it becomes a magical garden, home to the special fruit that is growing within it. In the early stages of pregnancy the placenta settles and attaches itself to the inside in the soft tissue of the uterus, putting out something like little roots and helping babies' bodies to grow.

Just imagine: no other muscle in the body is as well supplied with blood as the uterus, and the better the mother is supplied with haemoglobin, oxygen and all the important nutrients, the richer the nourishment that will pass through the blood to the uterus. Anything that arrives via the uterus will be filtered to be sure that only good things are passed on in the blood that goes through the umbilical cord to the baby – with the exception of certain sneaky substances like alcohol, which can cross the placenta with potentially damaging effects on the foetus. The blood runs through the baby once, and all the waste and the blood that has been used goes back through the cord into the muscle of the uterus and from there into the mother's body. Such a simple, yet amazing system.

The placenta is divided into two, with the maternal side attached to the inside of your uterus, and the upper side facing your baby. This side is covered with beautiful layers of tissue that form the amniotic sac, and that anchor the umbilical cord in its centre. The baby, floating in its bubble of amniotic fluid, is attached to the cord (I love the image of babies floating so effortlessly through time and space). At the end of your pregnancy you will have around one litre of amniotic fluid, which gradually begins to reduce.

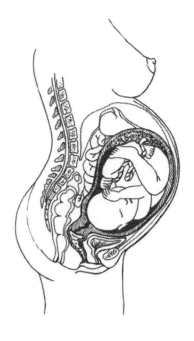

The baby floats in the amniotic fluid

When the waters start flowing...

In preparation for the birth, the amniotic sac will sometimes open up and release its fluid. Although birth professionals often speak of the 'rupture' of the membrane, it can be a very gentle moment. Some women may wake up in a puddle of fluid, others will just experience a constant dripping. The membrane can open up at any time before or during the birth, and this too will help the cervix to 'ripen' and get ready for the birth.

What happens next will depend very much on where you are. In Germany, for example, labour will be induced within twelve to twenty-four hours of the membrane opening. In Australia, where women come in for regular check-ups in the last stages of pregnancy, you will be left alone in the expectation that labour will start spontaneously within one to five days of the membrane opening. This makes more sense, as the majority of women do indeed go into labour of their own accord any time up to seventy-six hours after the release of the membrane.

The fluid should be a clear pinkish or very light yellow colour. If it is grass-green or mud-coloured, you need to contact your midwife or the hospital for a check-up. It needs to be investigated, but it may not necessarily stand in the way of a lovely natural birth.

For a midwife, the birth is only complete once the placenta has been delivered and all is well.

After the birth
Even once the baby is born, the placenta helps it to adapt to its new living conditions outside the womb. There is a reservoir of blood left in the placenta that, with each of the third stage contractions, will flow towards the baby, and then some will flow back. This gives the baby extra oxygen and a better start in life, and this process continues even when the baby is lying on your chest. For this reason the cord should only be clamped once its blood vessel has collapsed and there is no more pulse in it.

It's a bit like a mother holding her toddler by one hand, and only gradually withdrawing her support once he is walking steadily.

Once the placenta has been born, it's for the mother to decide what happens to it, but of course this varies according to customs around the world:

* In Australia and other places, some women practise lotus birth. This entails leaving the umbilical cord attached to the

baby until the placenta dries up and falls off of its own accord. This practice reflects the women's spiritual belief in the placenta as an eighth chakra (a chakra is a centre of spiritual strength in the body).

* This is not very common in Europe, where, instead, some women take a piece of the placenta and have a homeopathic remedy made out of it. They use this unique — you could almost call it bespoke — preparation when they feel sick or low in the postnatal period, or if the baby is not well. (In Germany, the home of classical homeopathy, special laboratories can prepare homeopathic tinctures or globules.) In my view it's a fantastic opportunity to make the most of the benefits of the placenta, but it's for you to decide.

* Some countries go for a more organotropic method called placenta encapsulation, which treats certain problems at a different energetic level. There are specialists who can undertake this, or you can buy placenta encapsulation kits. These make use of different methods: the Chinese medicine approach entails drying the placenta and placing the powder in capsules, or it can be processed raw and encapsulated.

* And in some cultures the placenta will be buried in the ground with due ceremony. In Europe parents might bury the placenta in the garden and plant a tree for the child above it. I learned when I lived in New Zealand that the Maori people bury the placenta with a special ceremony. This reinforces their strong association of the placenta with the land.

Our animal sisters usually eat their placenta, with the aim of protecting their babies from predators. And it's true that predators can usually smell blood and mucus, and this could alert them to the presence of vulnerable young prey.

Last, but certainly not least, I must tell you that in Germany we call the placenta 'Mother's cake'. I like that: it wouldn't really be a birthday without a cake!

Summary

Well, what have you learnt in Chapter 1? I took you through how birth really works, and how it can work for you. You now know about all the different hormones that contribute to the process of pregnancy and birth, and how they link sexuality to birth. We've explored labour: how it starts, how to encourage it to start, and to maintain it, what to do if it stops – giving you more control.

I know from teaching the contents of this chapter that people become excited at the prospect of their labour and gain faith in their ability to bring their skills to it.

In the next chapter I'm going to connect up some of the theory up with practical action that you can take to get your body in the best possible shape for the birth day.

Chapter 2: Happy birthing body

Instinctive birth and how to reconnect

Genetically every woman has the blueprint of how to give birth within her. You could see yourself holding hands with all women in an endless spiral extending from yourself, to your mother, your sisters, your grandmothers, your aunts, and their midwives — all standing close together, singing, humming and swaying their hips to the song of birth, the dance of labour. Even if you don't or can't have children, you are still part of this spiral, this sisterhood of women all holding hands and giving birth.

Birth as the start of life is the same the world over, connecting humans across the planet, whether you are a woman in Africa, India, Australia or Germany. The actual conditions and circumstances might be different, but the essence remains the same.

How can modern women in the digital age tune in to their instincts? Some might feel that they exist more in their heads than in their bodies; others might feel a bit lost and scared. For both there is the challenge of needing to look inside themselves and confront what will be expected of them at the birth. My message is simple: firstly, trust in your own abilities, and secondly, choose a place for the birth where you will feel safe, secure and understood. It's not a good idea to give birth in a place where people are incredibly busy and will look on you as just another woman.

So I advise you to trust your instincts, your gut feelings, and to enjoy this special time of your life, really allowing yourself to feel, hear and follow your own voice. Some women have incredible dreams about their baby and the upcoming birth.

Pregnancy can be a deeply creative time in your life: you are creating something so special that you might become as fertile on the outside as you are on the inside. Some women artists have told me that they have had an enormous flow of ideas around the time of their pregnancy, whereas others felt that all their creativity had been directed inwards to the womb, making it a magical place.

Anyway, feel free to indulge your fantasy, to connect up with your feelings in a free flow of energy and creativity. Some women choose this time to start writing a diary, others start singing, or painting or drawing. It's worth checking in with yourself to see if there is some old activity you would like to revive, or some new one you want to try. Do you want to get more into cooking, dancing, or yoga? Or do you want to take naps and explore the fertile land of daydreams that lies tantalisingly between waking and sleep? Whatever it is, you will want to watch out and see, feel and hear all that is changing within you.

Tip

Listen to the voice of your body as it leads you; the body that knows how to grow a baby also knows how to birth it.

We are all born with the ability to use our instincts and intuition at the birth —bear in mind that the body wants to give birth. The body that has been growing this baby for so many weeks knows exactly how to give birth to it, so we just have to go within ourselves and allow the mind and the body to connect deeply. Every woman possesses something we could call 'Internal wisdom', which can often be drowned out by medical knowledge and by all the activities that take place on the outside. Everybody has a voice, and every birth comes with a dream, a vision, of your baby.

Birth is still in effect a magical mystery tour, inviting you to take up the challenge of how to connect yourself with your body and the baby, but whatever happens, you will win the first prize.

Water: a powerful element

Water is the first element that humans are acquainted with. When we are in the womb, we float freely through time and space, entirely surrounded by amniotic fluid. No doubt at some level we remember dimly the ease and warmth of this fluid existence, since for most people water is very soothing and relaxing. How many of us like to wallow happily in a warm bath after a long day, or take a warm shower, releasing all our tensions and increasing our well-being? The image of floating in a beautiful pool sells thousands of holidays, tapping subliminally into our awareness that water calms the emotions and restores to us our sense of flow.

It was in the early 1990s that water births began to be accepted and to become more popular. I began working in an independent birth centre, the first one in Berlin to offer water births, and was amazed to see babies born into the water. In the years that followed hospitals had to follow suit because women demanded the comfort of a water birth. With the benefit of my experience I can endorse the effectiveness of taking a bath or a shower, or even giving birth directly into the water if that is what feels right for you.

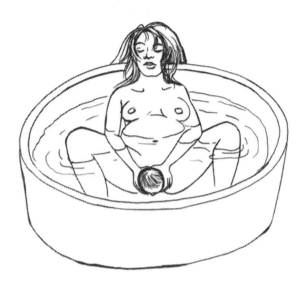

The comfort of a water birth

Whether you are planning to give birth in the water or not, it is very helpful to reach for the good old hot water bottle when labour starts and you feel the first contractions happening. Hopefully, most women will still have a hot water bottle at home! It can bring great relief, and can be placed wherever you are feeling the contractions. When you experience discomfort, it's a good idea to move around until you find the best position and to place a hot water bottle where relief is most needed. It may be simple and low-tech, but it works really well!

Once labour is progressing, you might want to take a warm shower, or hop into a warm bath. Even when I did my training in a large women's hospital in the south of Germany in the 1980s, we would invite every woman in labour to take a bath, just to get her more relaxed. I can't emphasise enough the benefits of water at this time. Even if you think it is not for you, I can assure you that just relaxing in a warm bath or on a birthing ball with a warm shower running can result in your cervix opening up amazingly.

Water in various guises really is the number one pain relief in labour. It was when I was working in Australia that I was really made aware of this. Many, many women asked for a bath to be run when they were admitted in labour. Some of them did not have access to huge amounts of hot water at home, so they enjoyed the unlimited amounts of it at the birthing centre. (Rental pools for a home water birth are absolutely wonderful, but if you live on an upper floor, you need to check that it will be strong enough to support a home birthing pool.)

Benefits of water labour and water birth

Research has confirmed the wide range of benefits offered by immersion in water during labour and birth.

Water:

* gives you mobility and allows you to get into any position you find comfortable during labour and for the birth

* speeds up labour

* reduces blood pressure

* gives you a greater feeling of control

* provides significant pain relief

* promotes relaxation

* conserves your energy

* reduces the need for drugs and intervention

* gives you a private and protected space

* reduces perineal trauma and the need for episiotomies

* reduces rates of C-section

* is highly rated by experienced birthing service providers

* encourages an easier birth for mothers and a gentler welcome for babies

* is highly rated by mothers, who typically state that they would consider giving birth in the water again, some even saying they would never give birth any other way

Placing a pool of water in a delivery room immediately changes the atmosphere: voices get softer, everyone becomes less stressed and the mother remains calmer.

The effect of buoyancy that deep water immersion creates allows the mother to move spontaneously. No one has to help her get into a new position. She moves as her body and the position of the baby dictate, and that movement helps open the pelvis, allowing the baby to descend.

When a woman in labour relaxes in a warm deep bath, free from gravity's pull on her body, with sensory stimulation reduced, her body is less likely to secrete stress-related hormones. This allows her body to produce the pain inhibitors – endorphins – that complement labour. Noradrenaline and catecholamines, the hormones that are released during stress, actually raise the blood pressure and can inhibit or slow labour. A woman in labour who is able to relax physically, is able to relax mentally as well. Many women, midwives, and doctors acknowledge the analgesic effect of water.

Movement skills to help your baby find the best position

Thousands of years ago, when we lived as hunter-gatherers, it was the women who were the gatherers. The job of gathering meant that women would walk, bend down, squat, pick or uproot something, stand again, and walk on. They would bend backwards and forwards to gather berries from bushes, and stretch up high to pick fruit from trees. They might have to kneel and dig strenuously with a stick to release tubers. All these movements, and others such as the rhythmical circular movements they would make sifting grain, would have helped prepare the woman's body for childbirth.

Modern women face challenges that simply did not exist for their foremothers. The whole of our lifestyle — how we eat, what we wear, and even how we think — can have a huge impact on our health, our emotional wellbeing and on the process of pregnancy and birth. We are likely to spend a lot of time in front of the television, relaxing on a sofa, or slumped in front of a computer screen, or driving. But you will remember that I highlighted this as a possible problem when it comes to getting the baby in the best position for birth. Midwives all over the world have put a lot of thought into solving the problem of babies being poorly aligned in the womb.

What you can do

But why is the baby's position so important, and what can you do to help your baby find the best position?

In the early weeks of pregnancy the baby floats freely above the pelvis. It moves and turns and rolls around, stretching its arms and legs in all directions. In the later weeks of the pregnancy it s in to more consistent contact with the pelvis, and takes up a position, though not necessarily its final position. It might want to curl up, head down, and lying on its side. If, for example, the woman leans back most of the time, perhaps while driving a car, or sitting at a desk, she could be sending a message to her baby that asks it to turn its spine towards the mother's spine.

This position is called a posterior lie, and it is possible for a baby to be born in this position, but it is much harder and takes much longer because the baby's head will be passing through the pelvis at an angle where it has a greater circumference. Women whose babies are in a posterior lie will experience strong back pains, sometimes feeling as though their back is breaking into pieces.

If the baby is not in the best position, women may spend many days in pre-labour as the uterus tries to correct the position. This is why it's so important to understand how your baby is currently positioned, and how you can help it to get into a good position. Don't hesitate to ask your doctor or midwife to feel for the position of your baby and give you a clear picture of how it is lying.

One really helpful technique is for women to spend a few minutes, several times a day, on all fours. When you do this, you are making your belly into a hammock and inviting the baby to snuggle up in the right way, with its head down and its spine turned towards your abdominal wall. While you're on all fours you could use the time to do a few rounds of deep or birth breathing, or you could put some pillows down and rest your head, or just have a drink and look at a magazine. Doing this at least two to four times a day, for just three to five minutes, will invite your baby to take up the best position — so kick off your killer heels, get down there and give it a go!

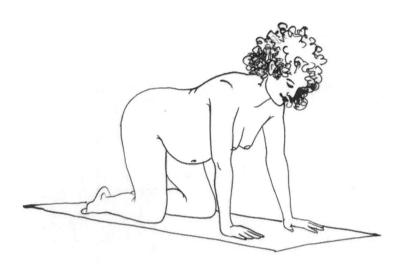

Make your belly into a hammock

The following exercises will also help you to tilt your pelvis in the right way to get the baby into the best position.

+ Stand upright and move your tailbone backwards and forwards, then bring it back to a natural position – don't have it sticking out in a 'ducky tail'!

+ Create a relaxed pelvic tilt by making a tight roll out of a small towel and placing it underneath you, so that when you sit at your desk, your pelvis is tilted forwards rather than leaning backwards, encouraging your baby to relax into the hammock.

Finally, get off your back! I'm all for rest and relaxation, but it's best for your baby if you can relax on your side, or at least with your upper body supported, leading your baby to snuggle into your belly. This goes for when you lie down to sleep at night as well. Use as many pillows or cushions as you like, but make sure you bend the knee that is uppermost when you are lying on your side, bringing it slightly to the front and supporting it with a pillow. This will make it easy, especially in the later weeks of your pregnancy, for your baby to find a great position to lie in.

Getting outside help

Sometimes our modern lifestyle – the soft mattresses we lie on, the shoes we wear, the positions we adopt while driving or at work – means that we find ourselves a bit out of alignment, and that we are simply not able to move things in the right direction by ourselves. Some women have a slightly tilted pelvis, or a very tight lower back, others have too much tension in the pelvic floor — all these conditions could encourage the baby to adopt a less than ideal position. If your tailbone is stuck or your pelvis is tilted, it will make it harder for the baby to get into the best position for the birth. That can create major problems during the birth. I get very apprehensive when a woman has a lot of really strong lower back pain, or great difficulty in walking.

If this is the case with you, see if you can find an osteopath, a gentle chiropractor, a Grinberg Method practitioner, or someone else who specialises in working with pregnant women's bodies to help release the pelvis or the iliosacral joint.

I have worked successfully with osteopaths for more than twenty years. Osteopathy is more than 200 years old and is a very gentle method to help your body, through gentle stimulation, to regulate itself. Each body has the ability to heal itself; sometimes it just needs to be reminded how to do so. Osteopathy is often combined with craniosacral therapy: this is a beautiful way to bring both the body and the nervous system back into alignment.

It is also a great method, after the birth, for helping babies to be well aligned, and I send most of my mums after C-sections, or long or difficult labours, to seek treatment for their babies.

Chiropractors are more common in English-speaking countries and some of them specialise in treating pregnant women – some will use an aid to gently align the muscles and the ligaments.

There are many different ways to bring about good alignment.

Looking after the pelvis

In our bodies everything is connected — the muscles to the bones to the joints. Joints are stacked above one another, and groups of muscles are connected and support the whole structure. The muscles that support your pelvis and the pelvic floor work together. But I have noticed that many more women nowadays suffer from inflammation of the pubic symphysis (the cartilaginous connection between the two sides of the pelvis). In this condition, the pubic joint loosens up and the pelvis distorts, leading to discomfort when walking, and possible sciatic pain. It is helpful for anyone who has this condition to strengthen the muscles that support the pelvis, bringing it back into the correct alignment.

If you think you have this condition, it would be a good idea to consult someone who can show you some exercises. Day to day, it's important to keep your knees together whenever you stand up. Opening your knees wide will aggravate this condition. This technique will not in any way impair your capacity to have a successful birth.

A useful exercise

This little exercise will help to strengthen the muscles in your pelvic girdle:

* Stand with your feet hip-width apart

* Put your hands on your hips and inhale Putting all your weight on your left leg, lift your right foot off the floor

* Keep your right leg straight and hold it a few centimetres of the ground

* Now bend your left knee as many times as you can, up to 25

* If you need a rest, have a rest, or do 10 repetitions at a time

* Take a rest and repeat the exercise on the other leg

Remember, just bend your knee a little bit: you don't need to go down very far to strengthen your muscles. If you do this exercise once to three times a day, you will feel the difference.

Finally, just walking for about thirty minutes every day will keep the big joints in the lower back moving and help your back to feel better.

How to prepare for avoiding a tear

Two of the main concerns that women have about childbirth are how to avoid the vagina tearing, and how to maintain the tone in their pelvic floor — the pelvic floor in particular is important both for controlling our bodily functions and for sex. As a general rule, nature does her bit and enables you to open up and give birth, but midwives from different countries have done a lot of research and conducted various trials to find ways to give nature a helping hand. There are also, of course, different customs from all over the world, drawing on traditional wisdom and knowledge.

The pelvic floor

The pelvic floor is a group of muscles that work together, keeping the base of the baby's 'house' strong during your pregnancy. As the pregnancy progresses the weight of the baby and the release of hormones combine to make the pelvic floor loosen and allow the baby to slide out into the world.

As a general point, being in good health helps your tissues to stretch. Make sure you have a healthy diet, to ensure that your muscles are well supplied with oxygen and nutrients. Good levels of haemoglobin in the blood mean that your tissues are in great shape and able to function effectively.

Practising pelvic floor exercises is also a key preparation — well-nourished and well-exercised muscle tissue will have the maximum amount of elasticity. With good muscle tone, you will be able to hold or release the pelvic floor at will, controlling the speed of the birth. Pushing the baby out with slow controlled movement is the best way to avoid big tears, as it allows your perineal tissue to stretch gently. The perineum is the area between the anus and the vulva, and it stretches considerably to allow the baby's head to pass through at the end of the birth.

The perineum

Doing a perineal massage from about thirty-six weeks into your pregnancy is a great way to start loosening up the perineum in preparation for the birth. You can do this yourself, or you can ask your partner to do it for you. Choose from natural oils that are made specifically for this purpose, or just use a wheat germ oil.

Whatever you go for, it should be a natural oil since this is such a delicate area of your body.

Your belly will be quite big by now, so it will probably be best for you to take up a semi-reclining position, putting a pillow into the small of your back to relax on. While gently massaging the whole perineal area, you can also insert the tip of two fingers into your vagina and just stretch the tissue slightly towards the anus. But of course, only do this if it feels OK for you. Some women find it helpful to imagine that they are greasing a small baking tin, and you may have other images that come to mind. Whatever works for you. And you only need to do it for five minutes a day.

The following exercise demonstrates just how effective massage can be at releasing and stretching tissues:

* Hold up both hands and touch your thumbs to your middle fingers. Compare the little triangle areas you have created.

* Now release your hands and start massaging one triangle area with the thumb of the other hand. Do this for a few minutes.

* Then hold your hands up again and create the triangle spaces: you will be surprised at how much bigger the triangle space in the hand that you massaged.

Some other useful techniques
* Take a steam bath or a bath in dried hay flowers

* In Germany some midwives use a warm cloth or a cloth with warm coffee on it to help to keep the perineum intact, and many women like the feeling of the warm soft pressure on the perineum.

* Some women take the homeopathic remedy coffea at c6 or c30 just before the birth.

* There is also an acupressure point on the perineum that can help.

Birth position

Finally, recent research shows that giving birth on all fours or in a birthing pool rather than while lying on your back reduces the risk of vaginal tears. Breathing the baby slowly down in one of these comfortable positions, or maybe while lying on your side or squatting, allows your pelvic floor and vagina to expand as naturally as possible.

Horse to lion breath: breathing your baby down and out

The importance of breathing during pregnancy and childbirth cannot be overstated! The influential Yogi Bajhan said that, 'Where there is breath there is life', and truly it marks the beginning of life. What is the first thing we do when we are born? We take a deep breath and fill our lungs for the very first time, then we exhale, and so the rhythm starts. From this very first breath at the beginning of life to the very last sigh as our souls leave our bodies (yogis believe our lives consist of a given number of breaths, and once these are used up we die), we breathe automatically, subconsciously.

Breathing should be like a river, running smoothly and freely, swelling when it needs to, and then returning to its usual rhythm. Breathing sustains us, we do it night and day, and while we might be able to hold our breath, we cannot stop it completely. And it's so much more than just taking in in oxygen. It infuses life into every step of our journey, including pregnancy and childbirth.

Breathing affects your respiratory, cardiovascular, neurological, gastrointestinal, muscular and psychic systems, so it is in effect the foundation stone of your life. Your breathing can tell you a lot about what is going on in your body, but you can also control it to support you and to help you relax and stay in tune for the birth of your baby. Through your breath you can enhance the well-being of your baby — even its growth — as well as support it during the birth.

The process of breathing

It has long been known that good breathing is one of the pillars of good health and of well-being. We know that if someone feels stressed-out and anxious, their breathing is usually fast and shallow. In such a situation the normal reaction would be to advise the person to take a deep breath and then to exhale slowly. And that's it: the sometimes-forgotten-but-thankfully-not-completely lost art of breathing!

Breathing lies at the centre of each action, and it can be a vital tool during birth. Though everything you feel and experience will influence your breath, knowing how to breathe well can help you to stay calm, to let go when you need to and can enable a positive birthing experience. Breathing is part of life support, and mothers can use effective breathing to help their babies feel good during the birth.

When you look at a newborn baby, you can see whole-body breathing in action, as breath is allowed to enter each part of the body. The whole body participates in the action of breathing. This is a capability we are all born with, yet most of us cease to use it as adults.

It is no surprise that breathing is an essential part of most bodyworks and body therapies, most notably yoga, Tai Chi and Pilates, but in many other disciplines and sports it's clear that coaches and students alike understand the importance of breathing and use it to enhance experience and performance.

So start off by observing your breath for a moment. Just feel it and notice if it's just going into your lungs, or deeper down into the abdomen, how long each part of the breath is, if it feels obstructed or if it is flowing freely. If you're under a lot of pressure, your breathing may become shallow and restricted, perhaps to the point where you no longer know how to release it. If you're out of breath, breathing with short breaths, or doing a lot of sighing, it's time to reconnect with your body and your breath. Become aware of your breath, and finally let it go.

Once you become aware of how you can improve the quality of your breathing, you will have knowledge of a technique that you can use for the rest of your life. By breathing life into every part of your body, you will feel refreshed and energised, yet still calm and relaxed. What's not to like?

How do I breathe?
You can do this simple observation by yourself or with a partner. Take a seat and make yourself comfortable. Allow your usual breathing to establish itself and then spend some time simply observing it. Don't try to change anything about it, just take notice of it.

* **Where to?** Where can you feel the movement of your breath most? Is it more in your chest, or more in your abdomen? More at the front of your body or at the back?

* **Where from?** As everything has an origin, try to identify where you think your breath originates.

* **Pace:** Is your breathing slow or fast? How many times to do you breathe in, in one minute?

* **Rhythm:** What sort of pattern does your breathing have? Are all parts of your breath equal? Is the in-breath longer or shorter than the out-breath? Do you pause at any part of the cycle?

* **Texture:** Are your breaths deep and resonant? Free-flowing or obstructed in some way? Are they consistent, or has anything about them changed during the period of observation?

Now relax and cease the observation. Once you are able to connect with your own breathing in this way, breathing for the birth will be much easier. It helps you to be in control, and to progress smoothly through the process of birth.

Building breathing for birth

Exercise One: three-part breath
This is a preparatory exercise for all the breathing exercises.

* Step 1: Place your hands gently on your belly, inhale through your nose and feel your belly expand, then exhale though your open lips. Repeat this three times.

* Step 2: Place your hands on the side of your ribs, and imagine that you are playing a harmonica, or even that you want to be Arnold Schwarzenegger. Inhale through your nose, feeling your ribs open up, then exhale through your open lips. Repeat this three times.

* Step 3: Place your hands on your chest. You might w
  picture your chest as a window opening onto the sky
  your heart shine out. Inhale through your nose, feeling the
  chest rising. (It will probably move a little less than your
  ribs and your belly did.) Again. Repeat this three times.

Through all these steps, the inhalations and exhalations should be
the same length, or you can double the length of the exhalations.

Exercise Two: horse breathing

Horse breathing is a great technique that can be used at all stages
throughout the birth. I learned it from a very old midwife and
have been using it for more than twenty-five years. Not only
does it help with the contractions, it's also extremely useful
during pregnancy if you are carrying a very small baby and your
placenta is not working well, as it will enhance your oxygen
intake, making it easier for the baby to grow and thrive.

* Inhale through your nose, hold your breath and in your
  mind count 21, 22, 23, 24, 25, 27, 28.

* Then exhale on a raspberry (which of course sounds like a
  horse) till your lungs are empty, hold empty counting in
  your mind 21, 22, 23, 24, 25, 26, 27, 28 as you do so.

* Inhale through your nose, hold your breath and in your
  mind count 21, 22, 23, 24, 25, 27, 28.

* Then exhale on a raspberry (which of course sounds like a
  horse) till your lungs are empty, hold empty 21, 22, 23, 24, 25,
  26, 27, 28 as you do so

* (It doesn't matter how far you count up, as long as the inhalations and exhalations are equal.

* Continue to do this until the contraction is over.

* When the contraction is over, relax your face and your body and keep them soft.

It may sound a bit strange, but give it a try. You never know when it might come in handy.

Exercise Three: doing the lion breath

Start off by standing or kneeling in a relaxed position:

* Roll your tongue and close your eyes.

* If possible with closed eyes look up to the place in between your eyebrows

* Then inhale, close your lips and swallow.

* Now, like a Maori warrior, move forward or bend your knees, open your eyes wide, stick your tongue out as far as it will go, and make a roaring sound: aaaaaaahhhhh-hhrrrrrrrrrr!

This exercise is great for to do in the early stages of pregnancy or birth. It is great for relaxing the face and jaw, and as these are connected to the pelvic floor, you will be relaxing the pelvic floor also.

Exercise Four: birth breathing

Birth breathing is to be used during the actual process of birth. In the following exercise, always remember to inhale through your nose and to exhale through your mouth.

This is what you do throughout the birth. You can practise this in bed with your partner at night or on your own.

* Imagine that you are a vessel and let your breath fill you from top to bottom.

* Closing your eyes, inhale though your nose – the air is going down in one long line to your baby, surrounding her with love and light, and then coming out in a soft exhalation.

* Continue to repeat these gentle breaths – each contraction will 'measure' about three to four of these long breaths.

* Once the contraction is finished allow your shoulders, face, lips and body to soften as your breathing returns to normal.

* As the next contraction begins, you start again straight away, breathing oxygen and love down and once round your baby, with a soft breath out.

* Inhale down though your nose in one line, and once around your baby, picturing a blossom opening, and exhaling a deep breath through your mouth.

* Once more inhale a sweet breath through your nose, down in one line, once around the baby with love and trust, and on the long breath out visualise everything that you want coming into being.

There is a birth breathing prompt sheet for you to copy and take with you on the day of the birth.

Be upstanding!

During the process of giving birth a woman must be free to choose at any time what feels best for her and her baby. Most of the time, when women are given this choice, they will choose an upright position. This could include bending forward, hanging on to a table, kneeling and using the wall as a support, or even using a rope hanging from the ceiling. The choice that offers most scope for movement is to hang on to your partner.

So what are the advantages of an upright position in childbirth?

A woman in labour often copes much better with all the discomfort and pain she may experience if she adopts an upright position. There are a number of reasons for this.

Emotional support

In this position it is much easier for the woman to maintain eye contact with her birthing partner — you will feel much more supported if you are looking into a pair of loving eyes that are willing you on, sending out the message, 'Yes, you can do it, just keep going.'

As midwife Naoli Vinaver said in her DVD *Birth Day*, a beautiful documentary about the home birth of her third child, 'When I was holding my partner's hands and looking into his eyes while walking forwards, it did not feel so much like pain any more. It felt more like our love that was growing in my belly, and as if our love, like the sun, wanted to burst out.'

 'No other natural bodily function is painful and childbirth should not be an exception'.

Dr Grantly Dick-Read

Women who are connecting deeply with the process of giving birth will benefit in many unquantifiable ways from being able to move freely.

The physical benefits

When the mother is upright, the baby can make the mo̶
natural gravity, descending more freely into the birth cana̶. ̶n
this position a woman may choose to make a swaying motion to
help the baby rotate down and out, just as some animals do. The
uterus is able to work more effectively in this position and, again,
the free flow that it allows sets up the right balance of tension and
relaxation that produces the result all interested parties are after.

It also seems that the flow of the blood to the placenta works
better when the woman is in an upright position as there is less
pressure on the placenta. This means there is a much richer
oxygen supply to the baby during the process of birth. Similarly,
a woman will experience less pressure on her diaphragm in this
position, and will be able to breathe more deeply, which will help
her to remain calm and oxygenated.

> ### Tip
> Sometimes it's good to rest, and sometimes you need
> to move.

The combination of movement and being in an upright position
seems to have a positive effect on the reticular activation system
in the brain, which helps the woman to stay more alert and
focused during labour, and experience less fatigue.

Women who experience great pressure on their lower back will
find great relief in in being able to get up and move about. The
five biggest ligaments that run from the iliosacral joint to the
uterus will have more freedom to stretch when the body is
upright or bent forward. Through adopting an upright position
and stretching up you can even help the abdominal muscles to

open up in a scissor-like motion, allowing the baby to slip into the pelvis easily, and then down and out.

All in all, upright positions and walking are associated with a shortened first stage of labour, and some studies have shown that they can reduce the need for an epidural in labour — a win/win situation for all concerned.

As ever, though, your gut instinct will be a good indicator of what's likely to work best.

Lock and key, or how to move the baby down and out

In an earlier chapter I explained the effect our modern lifestyles can have on the mother and the position of the baby. If the baby is poorly aligned, it can cause many problems in pregnancy and during labour.

Imagine one day you arrive home to find your door jammed. The more you bang on the door, the more firmly stuck it becomes, until you have to call a carpenter to come and release it. But if you had learnt how to 'swing and lift' your door to get it moving freely, you wouldn't have needed to summon help. This principle of 'swing and lift' works just as well for childbirth: the baby and the pelvis need to work together just like a lock and key.

I described earlier how hormones help to open the pelvis up, but the baby, with its ability to make its head smaller and to adjust the angle of its head to the shape of the pelvis, is doing its bit. The two fontanels in the baby's skull, one triangle-shaped and one diamond-shaped, allow the head to adopt a shape that will enable it to fit through the pelvis, and then accommodate the growth of the brain after birth. Nature is just amazing: she really wants babies to be born! Some babies are born with cone-shaped heads, but these go back to a normal shape and size a few days after birth.

Most of the time women have little awareness that they can open and close their pelvis, and yet they often instinctively move their bodies 'in a funny way' that is probably helping the baby to move through. So what could you do, consciously, to help your pelvis open up? First of all, you need to listen to your body and move it as it feels best. You will often end up automatically moving your legs and stretching micro-muscles in the right way.

But here's a little experiment you can do:

* Stand straight and bring your heels together, with your feet in a V shape.

* Place your hands on your buttocks and feel for your sitting bones. (If you have difficulty finding them, sit on your hands or your fists: you should feel two pointed bones in your buttocks. These are the sitting bones and they can demonstrate to you how mobile your pelvis is.)

* If you exaggerate the movement by bringing the knees together, you should be able to feel how the sitting bones are moving apart, demonstrating how the pelvis opens up like a beautiful bowl so that the baby can move into it more easily.

Many women quite spontaneously want to lean on a wall and turn one leg in. In this way they are natural creating more space on one side of the pelvis for the baby to wriggle down. Feel free to experiment with your feet and your heels. Turning your upper thighs in and out can also make a huge difference to your labour. Again, many women do this instinctively, but it's still good to try to feel how your body works, to get it into your cellular (and muscle) memory.

Another easy and effective way to help your baby move into the pelvis as your due date approaches is to walk up a long hill or up some stairs. The principle is always one of the rocking the baby down and into contact with the pelvis.

While you are actually giving birth it may feel good to bring one foot up on a little stool, or to use a Swiss ball (most birthing places offer one of these) in combination with a rope. Visualise yourself sitting on the ball, holding on to the rope attached to the ceiling and moving energetically from side to side and doing fast circular motions. Using the Swiss ball in this way feels really good, and you might even consider buying one for the home as babies love being rocked while Mum or Dad is bouncing gently up and down.

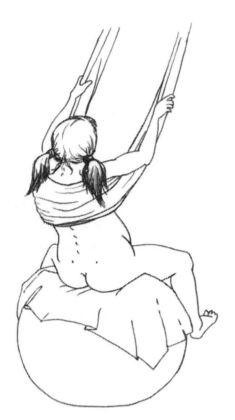

Upright position on a ball, supported by a sling to give maximum freedom of movement

Get dancing

Women often start circling their hips during labour. Circn...g your hips can help your baby to move, especially if it has got stuck somewhere. With your feet hip-width apart, take one step, imagining that you want to circle round the inside of your feet. On the next step circle round the outside of your feet.

Another very simple technique is to place your hands on your hips, or behind your head, and swing your hips naturally, as you would if you were dancing a samba. Not only is it fun, it- s great to practise in pregnancy because it helps to release the tension from your pelvis. All your birthing energy is in your pelvis, so if you want things to move, sometimes you have to move yourself!

Play around with your body and feel how you feel. This is an invitation to explore movement, breath and feeling. You are a beautiful woman enjoying this special experience for your body, and the baby will love being gently rocked in your womb. Babies learn many things inside the womb and, according to Dr David Chamberlaine, their sense of touch has already developed five weeks into gestation.

Let me share with you another technique I call 'Knee to Hip 1, 2, 3, 4' and give you an example of how effective it can be.

* Stand opposite your birthing partner and hold hands or the lower part of one another's arms.

* Look into each other's eyes and inhale.

* Starting with your right knee (always move opposite knees, as if you were dancing), bring your knee up as close as you can to your hip. As you inhale, think or say ' knee to hip

one', then on the other side 'knee to hip two... three' and so on, alternating the knees each time.

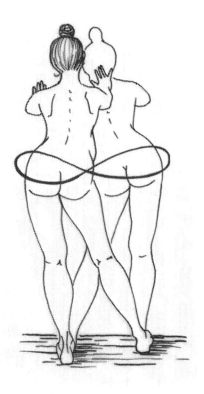

Case study: dancing to move the baby down

One day I was helping a woman who was doing really well. She got to the last stage of labour and was working really hard, but I could see from the baby's head that it was not moving down, no matter what she did. We tried all sorts of different positions, the birthing stool, etc. but nothing made any difference. Suddenly the 'knees, hips' exercise came to mind. I encouraged her to stand up and we did this exercise together for about thirty minutes, and in between, with each surge, she would squat down and move the baby further down and out – millimetre by millimetre, it seemed. Yes, it took a big team effort, but the baby was finally born, and the mother told me afterwards that she could feel the baby starting to move down once we started our knee to hip dance. You never know when your skills will come in handy.

This exercise is to be done during a break, not during contractions. The benefit of this exercise is that it enables your tailbone to move freely, which is a vital part of moving your pelvis. The tailbone should always be free to move, and not stuck on a soft mattress. However, don't do this exercise before 34 weeks, as you don't want to drive the baby deep into the pelvis in the early weeks of your pregnancy.

Case study: a damaged pelvis

Heather contacted me quite early in her pregnancy. She loved yoga and had joined my pregnancy yoga group at ten weeks. It was her first baby, and she had faced some serious difficulties in her life previously.

Five years earlier, she had been driven to jump from a railway bridge onto the tracks below. Somehow, she survived, but with major injuries, so she spent a year in and out of hospital, where her shattered pelvis was reconstructed, with 20 nails holding it together.

I wasn't sure what impact this would have on her pregnancy, but I encouraged her to keep coming to yoga and suggested some other treatments as well. I warned her that there was a 50% chance that she would have to have a Caesarean.

We worked with massage and acupuncture to stimulate the flow of energy in the pelvis, and we started work with hypnosis to release her fears and to focus on the development of the pregnancy and aim for as natural a birth as possible. Heather chose the well-known anthroposophic hospital in Berlin for the birth of her baby, and her pregnancy progressed smoothly.

Sometimes Heather worried about whether the baby would fit through her pelvis, but I reassured her that babies and their mothers are very clever, and mothers often manage to grow the baby to just the right size to fit through the pelvis. But I could see that Heather was still limping from her injuries, and I decided to send her to an osteopath, who would adjust her pelvis and get into a good alignment.

Finally the day of the birth arrived. Heather woke in the night with well-established contractions, her waters broke, and she made her way to the hospital, where she gave birth to a beautiful, tiny, healthy daughter; she was over the moon. The baby had to stay in the hospital for five days to ensure that breastfeeding was well established, that she was gaining weight, and that her blood sugars were stabilised. Heather, the baby and her partner all stayed in the family room, and all went according to plan.

I love Heather's story because I love stories that show how, with some knowledge, some preparation of the body and how to move it, and deep relaxation, what could have been a difficult birth experience became a positive one.

In touch with your partner

Note: Give this to your birthing partner to read, so they'll know what lies ahead, and what to do on the day!

It's your choice who you want to be with you at the birth of your baby. The touch and the mental support of your birthing partner are vital to helping you through the process of birth, so you need to think very carefully about who will be the best person to ask. It won't help you to have a birthing partner who is very unsure or anxious about the whole event.

Fathers have only been encouraged to be at the birth in the past 30 years, and who you choose will depend a lot on your culture, your relationship and your personal feelings. Keep your options open until near the end of your pregnancy, and consider whether you might want a friend, or your mother, or even a professional birth supporter as your back-up.

 'If I don't know my options, I don't have any.'
Diana Korte, journalist
and women's health campaigner

Having a supportive partner present at the birth makes the biggest impact when you are giving birth in hospital or at a birthing centre — if you 're planning to give birth at home, your partner is likely to be around anyway. In a hospital setting, it will make you feel safer and more supported to have with you someone who loves you, and who will be focused solely on all your needs.

Job description for birthing partners

Potential birthing partners need to understand that it's a full-on job, with little in the way of tea breaks. Mental and physical preparation are vital, as the birthing partner may be called upon to undertake a variety of roles: advocate for the woman, masseur, waiter, face-sponger, breathing guide — and they'll need to be sensitive enough to the woman's needs to identify which role they are being called upon to perform at any given moment. Wimps need not apply!

So what are the actual tasks the birthing partner may be expected to undertake on the day?

* Massage

* Setting the pace with breathing and holding the rhythm

* Supporting different positions in labour and keeping the pace

* Ensuring the woman feels strong and good about herself

* Running baths and preparing hot water bottles

* Helping the woman to stay focused on herself, the process of birth, and the baby

* Holding the space for her so she can open up and be herself

* Helping her to relax, find her voice and make sounds

* Offering drinks, nice food, dextrose and sips of energy drinks or water

* Reminding her to empty her bladder frequently

* Speaking a positive language

* Maintaining the cycle of breathing, baby breathing and resting between contractions

* Encouraging her to try different positions

* Being prepared to go along with whatever she wants at the time

* Asking for help, and

* Above all, giving her a feeling of being loved

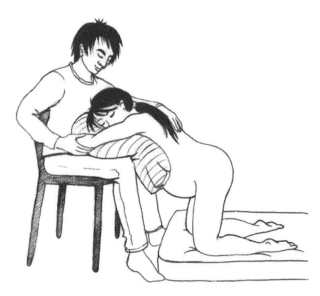

Supporting comfortable positions in labour

The woman and her birth partner are in this together, which is why it is so important that you discuss your plans and wishes for the birth with your chosen partner, so they will understand your choices, and so that you are both speaking the same language when the day comes.

Massage and breathing: a winning combination

As there are no absolute guarantees about how any given birth will unfold, it's a good idea to practise the breathing and the technique of a loving massage many times before the birth. Partners need to create a rapport during childbirth, and breathing and massage are non-verbal ways of doing so. We can communicate very well with our hands — often there is no need to speak, especially as sensitivity to non-verbal communication can be very high around the time of birth. It is exciting to be part of this silent story.

The basic massage is a very simple one: apply a natural oil onto the lower back and rub it in with a circular motion. Remember to include the hips and the tailbone area as these will benefit from a loving touch... You can massage with the palm or the knuckles of one hand, or with two. During labour, the focus is mainly on the lower back as there are five major ligaments connected to the iliosacral joint here, so this is where the woman will feel the sensation of pulling most intensely. Make sure you pack in your birthing bag a good oil that both of you like the smell of, as the massage may need to go on for several hours!

> **Tip**
>
> Find an oil that you like for your massage: lavender is calming and soothing; rose is beautiful during pregnancy and birth, and for the baby afterwards.

An effective way to get the most out of massage is to combine the rhythm of breathing and touch. The combination of deep breathing and slow movements while massaging the lower back is very effective, encouraging the woman to pace her breath with it, to relax and to stay focused.

Some women enjoy a firm massage, whereas others may prefer a softer touch. Sometimes just applying gentle pressure onto the sacrum towards the tailbone might be all that is wanted and needed, and in the later stages of birth women often enjoy a delicate massage of their inner thighs, or their shoulders or their face.

Your choice of birthing partner might also dictate which type of massage you feel most comfortable with. One effective technique is to massage, either with your fists or your hands, or still in rhythm with slow birth breathing, in a figure of eight across the lower back: what better way to show love and kindness to your partner?

Some women might not want to be touched at all... Luna unexpectedly gave birth to her first baby at thirty-seven weeks and withdrew so far into herself that every touch felt like an intrusion, an interruption of her concentration. Her partner was somewhat disappointed, as he had prepared carefully and was willing and eager to work with her, but she just said, 'I know what I am doing, it feels good and I feel fine,' and that was it.

Types of massage

Partner exercise
Practice this together in different positions to develop awareness and relaxation.

* Place your hand on a spot on her body, letting it sink in to it.

* Your partner then consciously breathes in to the spot where your hand is.

✳ Lift your hand gently and move it away.

✳ Your partner then just lets the feeling of touch at this spot melt away, taking any tension with it.

Some women may enjoy just having a warm hand or gentle pressure on their lower back.

Hands in motion

✳ Place one or two hands, palms down, on your partner's back. If you're using two hands, circle them in opposite directions.

✳ Breathe in rhythm with your moving hands.

✳ Move your hand(s) in big circles over your partner's hips and buttocks.

Practise varying this by easing the pressure as you breathe in and applying a bit more pressure as you breathe out.

Touch and relaxation

Gentle stroking with each slow inhalation and exhalation can help a woman to relax. You could do this kind of soft stroking on your partner's back, shoulders, or outer or inner thighs. It could also be a soft and loving touch of her temples, her forehead, or elsewhere on her face. What's important is to start practising this every day, whenever you catch your partner looking strained or tense. You can instantly remind her with a loving touch to 'let go'. If you practice this regularly in combination with the breathing, it can become almost like a reflex, and will happen spontaneously at the birth.

Gentle stroking (at one centimetre per second) is in fact a lifelong skill worth developing, as it stimulates the release of oxytocin, both in you and in the person you are touching.

Anyone can benefit: your child, your lover, an old person – and of course, your pet.

More, baby, more!

Once the baby's head is engaged and is moving further towards the tailbone, some women experience great pressure in their lower back, and may want to bend forward, circling their hips and pelvis, or they may enjoy firm external pressure to relieve it, or a very strong massage, demanding more and more depth to it.

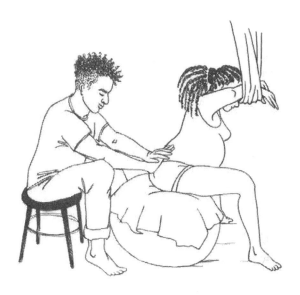

Some women may enjoy a very strong massage

I remember Gabrielle, for example, with each contraction shouting to her partner 'Stronger, stronger' in a loud voice while her partner worked really hard to support her and satisfy her. She really enjoyed making a noise, and sometimes yelled out 'Come, baby, come!' He told me afterwards that she felt as if the pelvis was having to stretch so much that it would break, and the firm touch and strong massage were the best relief that she could get for this. Never underestimate the power of touch.

Butterfly hands and the release of hormones

In our skin we have thousands of little nerves that act as transmitters. It is through this mechanism that touch releases oxytocin. This is why being touched gives us a feeling of connection, warmth, trust, and relaxation. An experiment by the Touch Research Institute in Miami has demonstrated that massaging muscles and skin has a calming effect on both adults and children: levels of the stress hormone cortisol may be reduced in a person receiving a massage.

So – what a useful piece of knowledge! Let's put it to good use:

* Stand behind your partner and take her spine as your middle line.

* Imagine your hands are like butterfly wings, touching only very lightly as in this case you want to activate the nerves, not work on the muscles.

* Place the backs of your hands gently on either side of your partner's tailbone and move them simultaneously up to the top of their head in a 'V'-like motion, covering as much space as you can, touching yet almost not touching.

* Once you reach the top of her head turn your hands over and let your palms gently flow down her ears, her shoulders and her arms.

* Then place your palms very gently on her shoulders and run

them down across her back in a figure of eight motion. This should feel as if she has four hands massaging her.

You can use this type of massage on all parts of the body, but in my experience it's most useful performed on the back during labour. Selena came into the birthing centre with her labour well established, ready to give birth to her second baby. She chose to stand, bending forward to lean on a cabinet while circling her pelvis, swaying her hips during contractions, and making a long 'Aaaahhh' sound. This worked really well for her, but her husband had to give a butterfly massage between contractions while she sipped on a drink and relaxed, and he had to do keep on doing this for some hours as this was all she wanted, until she finally gave birth while standing up. Her husband had practised many different techniques, but on this occasion only one was called for!

Tip

A study has shown that men can raise women's cortisol (stress hormone) levels at the birth, so make sure your partner is well prepared and knows how to support you.

The butterfly touch has in it an element of the soft exploratory touch of hands and fingers as a prelude to lovemaking, so you and your partner could take turns at it throughout your pregnancy.

Your birthing partner cannot know in advance what is going to be expected of them at the birth, but if they are well prepared, all options will be available. Above all, your birthing partner — be they the baby's father, your mother or your best friend —must be able to be sensitive to the needs of a woman in labour.

Many studies have shown that loving care and touch during childbirth can reduce the need for pain relief and leave women feeling that they have had a better experience. When we are touched with loving intentions it enhances the release of oxytocin, helping us feel connected and promoting the calming and pain-reducing effect that can help to make birth a special experience. Humans just thrive on loving words and a caring touch!

Hugs and kisses

Needless to say, sex and birth are closely related. Mostly you wouldn't be pregnant if you hadn't had sex! The hormones involved in these natural processes are the same, and it's helpful to know how to harness them during the birth.

The tongue and the lips are very sensitive parts of the body. When we kiss, the impulse runs through our nerves directly to our sex organs. Really intensive kissing can trigger a whole chain of chemical reactions in the body and enhance the flow of serotonin and endorphins, which make us feel both happy and really good. If kissing takes us to a greater level of excitement, this triggers dopamine and adrenalin, which will make us feel more positive, but also dull any pain, and lead to more of a pulsing sensation in the body, and finally to birth. So hugging and kissing — and I mean really kissing — are a great way to get all those lovely hormones going.

It might be quite helpful to kiss and hug between contractions. Sometimes labour slows down, even though you have had food and drink and a rest, and needs to be 'rebooted'. But if what you have been doing is not working, there is no point in just trying to do the same things harder. For example, if you have been moving about, squatting, standing and bending, and still nothing is happening, this might be the time to turn the lights off or down, and perhaps relax in a warm bath. Being in the dark will sometimes enable a woman to let go more easily.

Tip

Hugs before drugs: oxytocin not only helps birthing but makes you feel strong and unstoppable.

When you are relaxing in the dark, or in a semi-darkened space, all your other senses — smelling, tasting, hearing, touch — are triggered more easily, and you can use this to help you move the baby out more easily. Nipple stimulation can really help to get things going, and you could ask for some privacy so that you and your partner can kiss and massage lovingly and get things going again. Remember, sphincters and body orifices can become very shy when they are being ceaselessly poked and prodded and measured and stared at, which can lead to labour slowing down. Bringing some peace and privacy into the picture, and taking the pressure out of the situation, may well help to speed things up.

Living at the pace we do today can make it very difficult for us to accept that sometimes you just have to let go, accept the situation and stop trying so hard. So just allow things to unfold, without worrying about how longs it will take. Love and trust provide the foundation for giving birth, and you must trust that the love that brought your baby into being in your body will also help it to be born. You should understand that your body has grown, nurtured and protected this baby for all these months, and now your body knows perfectly well how to give birth to it. You can do it.

Shhhh! Birth in progress — do not disturb

Childbirth has become such a medicalised event in a woman's life that many of the medical practitioners involved in it have lost any understanding of the importance of leaving a woman who is giving birth undisturbed.

Most women, at least in the Western world, will choose to go to hospital to give birth. This has become part of our mainstream birth culture. What women often don't appreciate is that in fact they are going to an unfamiliar place to give birth, and they are likely to do so among total strangers.

The renowned midwife Ina May Gaskin has formulated a 'law of sphincters' that describes how the circular muscles in the uterus and vagina may respond to pressure: 'When a person's sphincter is in the process of opening, it may suddenly close if that person becomes frightened, upset, embarrassed, or self-conscious.' I agree wholeheartedly – our sphincters can react very strongly when we are shy, or feeling exposed or embarrassed in public. Think how often people become constipated when they go on holiday just because they are in an unfamiliar environment.

Birth itself is a very private act, just as making love is a private act. A woman needs to feel safe, secure and supported to open up. Shining a spotlight on her and constantly observing her are not the way to encourage her to do so. Looked at from this perspective, it's clear that a hospital birth can present quite a few challenges.

For a start, the woman giving birth, and the professionals surrounding her – the midwives and doctors – are approaching the big event from completely different directions. For the practitioners, the hospital is their familiar everyday working environment, one they feel perfectly comfortable in. For you, as the woman, it will be a strange place, yet one in which you will be expected to let go and open up in the most intimate way. How easy this will be for you depends a great deal on your cultural background.

I hope that this book will encourage midwives to be sensitive to this aspect of hospital birth, and to see themselves as champions of women and of normal birth, with a brief to intrude as little as possible. It is all too easy for professionals to become caught up in policies and protocols, and to lose sight of the realities that are evident to someone undergoing the experience for the first time. I therefore encourage you to speak up for your wishes and your rights at the birth. You might even get some long-serving birth practitioners to change their old, entrenched habits!

 'When you change the way you view birth, the way you birth will change.'

Marie Mongan, *Hypnobirthing*

The visionary obstetrician Michel Odent once said that the birth practitioner should sit in a corner and get on with some knitting. Remember, you can only give birth to this baby once, so this is your one chance to have a great birth. This opportunity should not be taken away from you by ignorance or intrusion. For both the woman and the midwife it is counterproductive if there is a level of disturbance that stops labour progressing. For a midwife, attending and supporting a birth that is flowing smoothly and progressing in its own time gives a feeling of great satisfaction that is shared by everyone involved.

This amazing process can be disrupted by any number of interventions in hospital: lots of medical examinations, constant timings and measurements, and beyond that simply to pressure to perform, to hurry up, expressed in words that, if not harsh, can be brusque and impatient. How can you be expected to open up, to reveal your vulnerability, in such a situation?

It is in an undisturbed environment that the hormones that enable birth will be released more readily. This may not necessarily mean that you will give birth more easily, but these hormones are indispensable to a good birth — the orchestra of hormones will perform in a more beautiful harmony if they can flow freely, without any disruption. So even in a hospital environment you should ask to be disturbed as little as possible, for examinations to be kept to a minimum, so that you and your supporters can create and maintain a peaceful and private atmosphere.

Some women will tell you that they felt as though they would have liked to withdraw into a private and protected space, like a little tent, to give birth. A friend of mine who opted for a home birth for her second baby created a small tent in her bedroom, and at a given point in her labour just crawled in there and went deep within herself to give birth. She had identified the need for a little private space for herself even in her own flat.

Wouldn't it be great if you could learn how to create that space within you no matter what your external surroundings? Well, I am going to do just that in a later chapter.

There is also a practical point to consider: if you have had an uncomplicated pregnancy, you should stay at home for as long as you can, until labour is well established. Your finely balanced hormones are more likely to end up out of tune if you move to the hospital too early and start to feel under pressure to perform. Most midwives agree that it is normal for labour to slow down once a woman arrives at hospital, only to pick up again once she has made herself at home there. In Chapter 8 I will also give you some hints and tips about how to do just that, but just for starters it's not a bad idea to put up a 'Do not disturb' sign or asking people politely if you can be left alone as far as possible. Just a little bit of preparation can make a big contribution to a great birth.

Remember, birth is even older than humanity, so she knows very well how the process should unfold, and we should honour that.

Making the right noises

Giving birth to a baby can be so fantastic that sometimes we give voice to a sound that comes from deep within. Many women have told me after their babies were born that at some stage they just could not help it, they just had to let a sound come out. And they were often surprised at the quality and richness of the sound that came out. Making a sound can be very helpful, but your willingness to go with this will depend a lot on your culture, and also on what sort of person you are.

It's useful to be aware of the different ways you can benefit from making a sound. We all know that sometimes when they are making love men and women alike make sounds and that these just slip out naturally. This could also happen during childbirth: a sound might just want to free itself along with the baby, and giving in to this urge will help you to let go and open up to deliver the baby.

That's why it's worth understanding how you can direct sound and use it to relax your belly, your pelvic floor..., and your jaw. When I first started out, in midwifery school, I learned that when ᴸower jaw is relaxed the pelvic floor is relaxed. Since then I have observed how some women want to shout things like, 'come, oooohhh baby, come!', while others just relax while emitting a long aaahhh, ooohhhh, or uuuhhhh, or even eeehhh.

Focus on the jaw and the pelvic floor

This exercise comes from yoga and is very helpful for releasing the lower jaw as well as the pelvic floor.

* First relax in a semi-reclining position, put your thumb in your mouth and start sucking on it vigorously. Put your other hand on your pelvic floor, and you should be able to feel a motion in your pelvic floor. Next, either staying where you are or getting to your feet, and tighten up your face as much as you can. You will be able to feel how your pelvic floor tightens up. Repeat this a few times, relaxing between each cycle.

* Now either roll your tongue at the tip, if you are able to do that, or if not, purse your lips up as if you were about to kiss someone, inhale deeply, close your lips, swallow, then open your mouth. Stick your tongue out as far as it will go, open your eyes wide and let a roaring 'Aaarrrggghhh' sound come blasting out... you are a lioness! Keep on doing this a few times and notice how relaxed your jaws become. This is a great little exercise to perform if you feel you need to create more space and a feeling of greater relaxation on the pelvic floor.

* This exercise could be followed by a directed sound to support the pulsing movement of labour and to help you harness the energy to move the baby down and out: feel the different qualities of the vowel sounds aaahhh, eeehhh,

ooohhh and uuuhhh. I think 'eeehh' is the most constrained sound of all of them, but it has the advantage of making you smile to produce it. The other sounds remind me more of an alpenhorn, a didgeridoo, or a big flute, allowing the sound to be directed accurately to shift both the discomfort and the baby!

All these exercises can seem a bit strange when you are doing them as a dry run, but persevere with practising them at home, and you will soon get used to them.

The power of song

In my yoga for pregnancy class we usually finish off with singing at least one song. I encourage singing at all stages of pregnancy as I believe everybody has a voice, and it can be very helpful to know how to use it. When you sing, you breathe more deeply, and if your body is flooded with oxygen, it finds it easier to let go.

As we know, singing fosters togetherness, and many cultures express this through their traditions and customs. When you sing you breathe, and this breathing is focused on one purpose, keeping the mind from wandering to unhelpful thoughts. There is a TED talk about a man who sang every day for ten minutes, and he noticed that this was helping him to feel happier and more positive about life. Similarly, singing and humming during pregnancy help to build more happy hormones in the brain, which is a great investment for the birth itself.

Here is another exercise, this time from my singing practice, designed to help shift things: place your hands on your hips and exhale while saying 'Shuft, shuft, shuft, shuuuffftt... YEAH!' Now inhale, and with each exhalation make a long sound while you relax your jaw, tuning in to what feels best for you right now.

Just imagine being a baby and floating around in a beautiful pool of water, gently rocked to and fro by the pull and the vibration of the fluid. Babies love it when their mothers make sounds and sing. They can hear from around the fourteenth week of pregnancy, and become attached to the sound of their mother's voice. This is the sound of love and trust, so when you sing or hum, or speak, or in fact make any sounds it makes the baby feel good, and will allow you to let go more easily.

On days when you are feeling vulnerable, or if you just enjoy doing these kinds of exercises anyway, you can stand, sit, or kneel and imagine that with each inhalation you are inhaling light, harmony, and good feelings. When you exhale, make a sound — a hum, short or long, soft, or growing volume like a wave, or a smooth monotone — and as you do so imagine that you are building a protective structure around yourself layer by layer: a bell or an igloo of sound, to protect you and make you feel good.

Blood, sweat and tears: why every woman is a winner

The end game

At long last, it's your birth day! As they think about the last stages of the birth, and can feel the baby start to move, women may become anxious and uncertain, or feel that they will just not be able to get the baby out. It's important to remember that, no matter how she finally gives birth, every woman is a winner and deserves to feel like one as well.

Sometimes things don't turn out as you expect: I can't deny that between 8% and 11% of women will need a C-section or some other sort of assistance. No matter how well prepared you are, there is always the X factor, the unknown element. The wind may shift at any moment, and you have to be flexible and go with the flow. Above all, it's important to resist the feeling that you may not have done enough. I am convinced that all women give of their best, in the context of their own knowledge of their bodies and of the prevailing circumstances. So I raise my glass to them, as that is definitely something that should be honoured.

It makes me sad that a competitive element has entered even this area of our lives. It's not about who has had the better, faster, most natural, etc. birth. Just bringing another being into the world is very special.

Coping with a crisis

Even if things don't end up going the way you want them to, you can still use your preparations to calm yourself in the face of uncertainty and anxiety, and make the most of any situation, as the following story illustrates.

Case study: deep breathing

At the birthing centre I worked with a couple who were well prepared and who were hoping for a natural birth. Louisa was sitting in a bath tub, the atmosphere was calm and serene, and all looked set fair for the birth they had in mind. But when I checked the baby's heart rate, I could hear that it was dropping down very low, and taking a long time to recover to a normal rate. I checked a few more times at frequent intervals, but there was no improvement; if anything it was getting worse. We tried a few techniques to improve the baby's heart rate, but it was clear that they were not making any difference. I explained my concerns to Louisa, and asked if I could examine her cervix, to see if there was any prospect of the baby being born fairly soon.

Unfortunately her cervix was only four centimetres dilated, so there was no birth in sight yet. I had to transfer Louisa to the labour ward, knowing deep inside that if things did not improve we might have to go for a C-section. In the labour ward I handed Louisa over to the care of the obstetric team, but I stayed with her for support, and to help her with her breathing. We followed the birth breathing, and every time the baby was in distress, Louisa's deep breathing at least brought its heart rate up a bit quicker. This did not alter the fact that time was running out, and finally we had to go for a C-section. The surgeon lifted out a small, sweet baby boy, completely tangled up in the umbilical cord. There was simply no other way in which this baby could have been delivered.

We were all grateful for the safe delivery of this little boy, and this birth showed me yet again how much good breathing can help: it might not guarantee you the birth you wanted, but it can still be supportive and help you to stay calmer in the face of emergency.

Louisa had got practically everything she didn't want, but at the end of it all was still holding a beautiful baby in her arms. So that is why I think every woman is a winner.

After the birth: the undisturbed golden hour

Hooray! You have done it, and that is something that should be honoured. Once you are holding your baby in your arms, you should feel free to enjoy the sense of achievement, and to give rein to your emotions. Whatever you experienced during pregnancy and labour will be worth it once you feel that little body resting on your chest and snuggling up to you.

Now is the time to enjoy a moment of privacy, and it's good for the couple to be left alone to savour this magical moment. Undisturbed skin to skin contact between mother and baby will enhance the release of oxytocin. The oxytocin levels of newborn babies peak at around thirty minutes after birth, and mothers will experience a peak at around sixty minutes after the placenta is born. This is the golden hour that mothers, babies and partners should revel in: mothers and their babies are floating in an amazing cocktail of hormones and emotions. This moment will never come back, which is why it's worth asking the staff at your hospital or birthing centre to allow you some time and space to appreciate it fully.

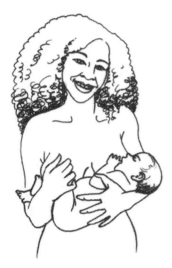

Skin to skin contact

This is also the time to get acquainted. While animal mothers usually lick their newborns, human mothers usually cuddle, kiss and stroke their new babies very gently and lovingly. The babies themselves are born to be very alert, and to participate in this moment. All their senses are wide open, and they are attuned to survival. Babies want to be born, and they also want to live.

Licking, nuzzling, and finding the breast helps babies feel good, safe and secure. Through the closeness to their mother they can smell, feel, hear and understand that this is their mother, the person on whom they will depend for their survival. It is through their senses that mother and baby recognise each other.

It is because of their sense of smell that babies are attracted to their mother's nipple, and their instinct is to try and crawl up to the mother's breast to feed —nature is amazing! It's important to understand this, especially if you end up having to have a C-section, because you will need plenty of skin to skin contact with your baby to get the oxytocin flowing. There will be plenty of time to weigh and dress the baby later, after the baby has had its first feed and the crucial bodily connection between you and your baby has been established.

Leading oxytocin researcher Kerstin Uvnas-Moberg has discovered that oxytocin acts as an effective anti-stress agent, lowering fears and anxieties. In her research she demonstrated that mothers who breastfed for more than seven weeks were calmer by the time their babies were six months old than mothers who had not breastfed at all.

Tip
The bed in the birthing room is a great place for bonding with your baby after the birth

As a midwife, I feel it is a special privilege to be present at the birth of a baby, no matter how many mothers I attend. Being the gatekeeper of birth for the mother, the father and the whole family has always been, and continues to be, a great honour.

So I speak from my heart when I congratulate you and urge you to enjoy this precious moment in time, holding your priceless gift in your loving arms.

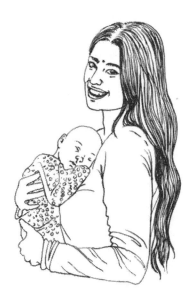

Summary

In Chapter 2, we focused on your body. We travelled from breath to touch, and I explained how they are connected and can be used in different ways. You can start doing the simple but effective exercises right from the beginning of your pregnancy, including your partner in the breathing exercises so they'll know what to do on the day – you can even do this as you lie down together at night in a spoon position! Your partner has an important job to do on the day, so now is the time to build on the rapport between you.

Preparing the pelvis is vital, and I have shown you how to help your baby into the best alignment for her journey through the pelvis by moving and resting in the right way. What better way to connect with your baby?

The birth stories tell of how you can use techniques whatever happens, to help yourself and to help your baby.

Chapter 3: Happy Birthing Mind

'Lose your mind and come to your senses'

This quote from Fritz Pearls, the father of Gestalt Therapy, supports my view that it is just as important to set your mind in the right direction for childbirth as it is to get your pelvis into the right alignment.

Your mind is capable of creating limits on how your body can act, so let's harness the mind's power to expand both your outlook and your body for the benefit of your pregnancy and birth.

I've already flagged up that birth is a primal act, and therefore our knowledge of it is instinctive. Instinctive behaviour comes from deep inside our subconscious and shapes our actions and reactions. During pregnancy many women instinctively talk to their babies and see them from the beginning as a real person. This connection with the baby and with your body can be enhanced through relaxation, mind and body work, yoga, hypnosis — and even just through touching and stroking your belly.

So what kinds of preparations do we make for birth these days? The image most women have of childbirth is highly coloured by television, film, and stories in magazines, and it is often far removed from the truth. As we rarely attend births, and don't live in big family communities where we would get a chance to see for ourselves at first-hand what the experience is really like, we have to piece together a lot of rather unsatisfactory information and usually end up dwelling on an anecdote about a friend of a friend who was in labour for days and then ended up having to have a C-section.

High drama is a bigger draw than a beautiful, peaceful and natural birth, and this means that a lot of women are full of fear as their due date draws close and their courage begins to fail. But I can't emphasise enough the importance of working on your mind to help you achieve a good birth. Just as Martin Luther King had his dream of racial harmony, I have a dream that one day every woman will have the opportunity to achieve a joyful and safe birth for her child, no matter the setting in which she gives birth.

> ## Tip
> Surrender, surrender, surrender: a doctor once said that the best medicine for humans is love. Someone asked, but what if this is not enough? The doctor said, just increase the dosage.

This chapter should be like the key in the door to a beautiful birth. We live in exciting times: science has generated computers and space travel, but it has also been able to reveal to us much about how the brain works. Birth has been around for a long time, and it works in exactly the same way as it did when we first started walking upright on the face of the planet. So why do we now feel that it is an immensely complicated process?

Part of the reason is that we seem to have become obsessed with the problems that can occur in pregnancy and childbirth to the exclusion of everything else, and this has led to stress. Whenever you feel anxious or insecure your brain will produce a huge number of stress hormones. This is all very useful when you need to run for your life, but decidedly unhelpful if you want to have a joyful pregnancy and a positive experience of birth. What's more, if you are highly stressed out over a long period of time, you might end up burnt out, whereas this is the time to blossom and relax.

Stress and fear are the enemies in the birthing room, and the earlier you can dispel worries from your mind the more joyful your pregnancy will be, and the calmer your birth. If the fight or flight response is triggered during labour, it can lead to the vicious circle of fear leading to tension pain, which of course only leads to more fear and increased tension pain. This can stop the production of birth hormones and cause some really unwanted outcomes. (What's more, babies don't like stress either: a high number of stress hormones present during pregnancy can lead to a lower birth weight.)

 'Giving birth should be your greatest achievement, not your greatest fear.'
Jane Weideman, founder of Birth Buddy

This is the time to draw on the knowledge in the earlier chapters about harnessing the power of hormones, and using breathing and touch to release oxytocin that will calm your anxieties, and endorphins to make you feel good.

The power of hypnosis

It has probably never occurred to them, but most women probably spend their pregnancy in a state of negative hypnosis. Every thought leads to a biochemical reaction in the body, so we need to use this information to counter this negative hypnosis and get the brain set up to generate good feelings and helpful hormones.

Ever since I first went for hypnosis many years ago, I have never lost my interest in, or trust in, this method. It works because our amazing brains work a bit like a computer: sometimes we find that a Trojan has taken it over and is supplying us with false information, but all you need to do in this case is overwrite the software in your brain.

So let's get started with some relaxation and techniques for creating and maintaining good feelings within you. Find a partner or friend to read this exercise out to you, or you could record it on your phone, or even memorise it.

✳ Start with slow breathing: inhale through your nose, counting 1, 2, 3, 4, 5 and exhale slowly through your open lips, counting 1, 2, 3, 4, 5, 6; inhale gently 1, 2, 3, 4, 5, and exhale gently 1, 2, 3, 4, 5, 6 — a long, soft breath in and a long deep breath out.

✳ Keep your eyes closed, your lips relaxed and your shoulders soft.

✳ Now think about a happy moment in your life: see yourself in a happy moment, see your happy face and hear the sounds that are around you.

✳ Once you have got an image, bring the thumb and the middle finger of your hand together and start tapping them, while you make the image in your mind bigger, brighter and more colourful.

✳ Once you have reached life-size, jump right into yourself and see what you saw then, hear what you heard then, and feel the feeling of feeling happy, and when this feeling is at its peak, squeeze your thumb and middle finger together as hard as you can to anchor the happy feeling. Release your fingers and take the good feeling into the next round of breathing with you.

✳ Again, with your eyes closed, inhale gently through your nose, counting 1, 2, 3, 4, 5, 6, and allowing the breath to fill your body with feelings of light and harmony; exhale a long, soft breath through your lips, counting 1, 2, 3, 4, 5, 6, 7; take another soft, effortless breath in 1, 2, 3, 4, 5, 6, 7, and release a long deep breath out 1, 2, 3, 4, 5, 6, 7, 8. Repeat this one more time.

* As you do so again visualise the happy moment in your life, making the image even larger and more colourful, squeezing your thumb and your middle finger together as you listen again to what you heard and feel what you felt at the time.

* Now think about a relaxed moment in your life; see yourself in a moment of total relaxation, and see the colours and hear the sounds that go with that moment. Now bring the middle finger and thumb together and tap them as your make your picture bigger and brighter.

* When you reach life size, jump into yourself and see what you saw, hear what you heard and enjoy the feeling of being so relaxed and so soft. Squeeze your middle finger and thumb together to anchor this wonderful feeling.

* Again, with your eyes closed, inhale gently through your nose, counting 1, 2, 3, 4, 5, 6, and allowing the breath to fill your body with feelings of light and harmony; exhale a long, soft breath through your lips, counting 1, 2, 3, 4, 5, 6, 7; take another soft, effortless breath in 1, 2, 3, 4, 5, 6, 7, and release a long deep breath out 1, 2, 3, 4, 5, 6, 7, 8. Repeat this one more time.

* And one more time, see yourself in a joyful moment of your life. See yourself smiling and laughing, and bring your thumb and middle finger together and tap them, as you make the image bigger and brighter.

* Once you reach life size, jump into yourself and see what you saw and hear what you heard at that time, enjoying the feelings of ease and joy. Squeeze your middle finger and thumb together to anchor this wonderful feeling.

* Again, with your eyes closed, inhale gently through your nose, counting 1, 2, 3, 4, 5, 6, and allowing the breath to fill your body with feelings of light and harmony; exhale a long, soft breath through your lips, counting 1, 2, 3, 4, 5, 6, 7; take another soft, effortless breath in 1, 2, 3, 4, 5, 6, 7, and release a long deep breath out 1, 2, 3, 4, 5, 6, 7, 8. Repeat this one more time.

Repeat this easy-to-follow exercise at least three to five times, and you will be amazed at the difference it can make. Whenever something nice happens in your life, just squeeze your thumb and middle finger tight and anchor the good feeling. In this way squeezing your middle finger and thumb together will evoke those good feelings. These anchors really want to be used!

Circle of life breathing: relaxation

This exercise will also help you to prevent negative thoughts and achieve the birth you want, but it is useful at any time when you want to relax quickly:

* Breathe in and out calmly, imagining that you are inhaling positive energy through your nose.

* Imagine this positive energy flowing smoothly down the front of your body.

* This positive energy is filling your chest, arms, your belly, your legs...

... down, down, right to the tips of your toes.

* As you exhale, the positive energy flows all the way up the back of your body.

* You can feel it moving gently up from your heels, up the back of your thighs, your buttocks, all the way up your back to the top of your head, until your head is filled with positive energy.

* Now gently inhale and repeat the process.

Use this technique any time you want to get yourself into good state of relaxation. It's important to know how to stop the spiral of thoughts, and with this method you can open the gate to your subconscious and introduce some positive thoughts. Did you know that you can actually chat to your subconscious and introduce some positive thoughts into it.

Visualise all you want

Your mind is like a library, a video store, and a museum all rolled into one, and you can fill it with good things that will help you to realise your wishes, becoming your own Dr Feelgood, the curator of your collection. Dr Feelgood will harness your inner resources, drawing from the outside world and your interior world; she will also spot the things that might prevent you from achieving your goal. Here is one of her prescribed exercises:

* First control your breathing, to gain a state of calmness.

* Picture a big screen; if a negative thought comes along, imagine a big 'stop' sign coming along to obliterate it.

* Imagine something positive like love or happiness spreading across the screen, contained in a really vivid colour; 'see' it at least three times.

* Now watch the 'positive' footage of yourself as you relax deeply into each contraction; feeling soft and open as the birth progresses.

* You could even picture your surprised face when you realise the baby has slipped into the world almost unnoticed; you look up at the clock in amazement.

* See yourself as you pick up your baby for the very first time and gaze into its eyes – make the picture as vivid and defined as you can.

* Enjoy the feeling, and let it become bigger and stronger, moving through your body and filling up your mind. Believe that you can do it.

Dave Elman's method and why you should understand how to use it

Dave Elman's 'induction' method of rapid hypnosis has been famous for over 60 years. He witnessed the magic of hypnosis as a child, when his father, Jacob, was very ill with cancer. A friend came to the house to give him a hypnosis session for pain relief that was effective enough for Jacob to be able to play with his son again. Dave was so impressed that he began learning these techniques from the friend. In 1949 he began teaching his technique to doctors and dentists.

Below is an adjusted version of the Dave Elman method that I love. It works well, and I use it for many things in my own life. It's great to use this technique, or parts of it, to help you go deeper and deeper into a profound relaxation. Practice following the instructions below a few times, and once you have done it a few times, it will be easy to use it whenever you need it.

* Gently close your eyes.

* Focus on the small muscles to the right and left of, and all around, your eyes. Imagine them all starting to relax.

* Keep on relaxing these small muscles; you will noticed that the more relaxed these small muscles round your eyes are, the more tightly closed your eyes will be.

* You are so relaxed you couldn't open your eyes even if you tried; it feels so good to finally relax.

* Sink into your ideal of deep, endless, soothing relaxation.

* Start counting down from 100 in your head, and with every number double the relaxation until the numbers just float away and you forget all about them.

* Give yourself permission to relax this deeply.

* Your mind and your body are completely relaxed; you have taught yourself how to relax them on the day of the birth.

* Now try to open your eyelids.

Don't worry! Your eyelids won't be closed for ever. This also works the other way round: if you just imagine the muscles round your eyes are tensing, gaining energy, you will be able to open your eyes easily.

You can use this 'induction' method in different ways: to relax, to fall asleep, and to teach yourself to trust in your own bodily skills. Following the instructions above, once your eyelids are tightly shut, tell yourself that your body knows very well how to birth your baby, and the birth will come to you effortlessly and easily.

If you feel any resistance to this method, or doubt about whether it works, continue to practise it, telling yourself that every day you feel better and better, and that you trust your body to know what to do.

Creating the right feelings...

... and by that I mean good feelings, of course! There is a saying in Buddhism: 'If you have a problem, why worry? Either you have the solution to the problem, in which case there is no need to worry, or there is no solution to the problem, so worrying will not help to solve it.'

What we think about, what we have on our minds every day, makes a huge difference to how we feel, so training your brain to generate good feelings throughout your pregnancy will help you to reach out for those feelings when you are in labour.

'You've gotta dance like there's nobody watching,
Love like you'll never be hurt,
Sing like there's nobody listening,
And live like it's heaven on earth.'
And give birth exactly this way...

William W. Purkey

Your brain does not make a distinction between a fake smile and a real one, or between fake laughter and genuine laughter. All it registers is that you are laughing and smiling. Well, now's the time to put such trickery to good use.

Laughter, the best medicine

Laughing, even for no reason, is extremely constructive, and for many years now people have been joining laughter yoga clubs and schools all over the world. Dr Manda Kataria is well known as the Giggling Guru, the Laugh Doctor, and he says 'Laughter is universal: it does not know any language or borders, it does not make any difference between castes, beliefs and colours. It is a powerful feeling and has the ingredients to unite the world.'

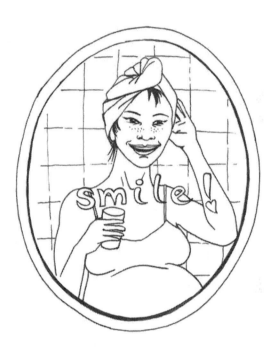

According to scientific research, children laugh around 400 times a day, whereas adults only do so around 15 times. Many women seem to be under a lot of pressure during their pregnancies, dwelling on the stress of what might happen next rather than enjoying this very special time in their lives. Time to cheer up, I think.

It might surprise you to know that laughing for just 10 to 15 minutes a day can change the chemistry in your brain and the way you feel.

So:

* Remind yourself to smile as often as you can throughout the day.

* When you look at yourself in the mirror in the morning, wave, smile a big smile at yourself and yell, 'Hey, I'm back!'

* Pay yourself a compliment, such as, 'Wow, my belly looks fantastic!'

* Just start laughing, whether you're standing, sitting or lying down. If you find this hard to do, just try inhaling and then letting your breath out on a 'hahahaha' sound. Then carry on with a 'hohoho' and a 'heeheehee'. It works, and the only way you will find out is by giving it a go!

Gratitude

Another beautiful and very simple exercise to develop these positive feelings is the exercise of gratitude. Every morning when you wake up just take a moment to remind yourself of something that you are thankful for. This could be anything, no matter how small: a funny text from a friend, the comfort of your pillow... find at least three things.

Then, when you go to bed at night, think back over the day and find three to five things that you enjoyed, that made you happy, that you are grateful for. This is a great way to book-end your day, and to start anchoring these positive feelings and making the most of them.

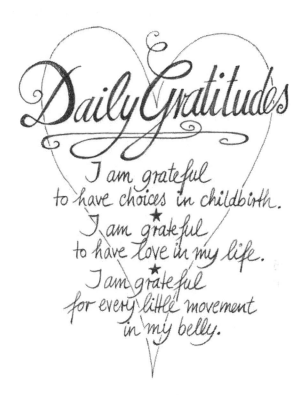

Daily Gratitudes

*I am grateful
to have choices in childbirth.
I am grateful
to have love in my life.
I am grateful
for every little movement
in my belly.*

Finding your focus

There is great truth in the saying 'what you resist is what persists'. If I were to say to you, 'Don't think about a blue elephant covered with pink spots', you would instantly find a large herd of such beasts stampeding through your mind swinging their trunks flamboyantly... even though I had expressly asked you not to think about them. Whatever you are focusing on is what will stay in your mind.

Another example: look around the room you are in right now and pick out all the red things. Now close your eyes and recall all these red things. Now, still keeping your eyes closed, recall all the blue things... How did you get on? No doubt you did well at recalling the red things because this is what you had been asked to focus on.

 'In order to succeed, we must first believe that we can.'
Nikos Kazantza

Here is another exercise that you could do by yourself or with a partner. I learnt it when I went to a beautiful school in the north of England in 2005 to study hypnosis and hypnotherapy. My teacher was Will Proudfoot, an enthusiastic octogenarian, and I have fond memories of his skills and of the experience of training with him. There is a great method called Focusing and you can find the words and the exercise for free on the internet. Focusing is a 6-step method that has been developed by Eugene T. Gendlin.

Let me share a beautiful and simple exercise that might take you by surprise. But as I have learned through my work, not only is it helpful to change the quality of the pictures, the movies in our head, it is worthwhile working with our emotions as well. In 1950, a big study in Chicago showed that people, no matter what problem they had, no matter what type of therapy they used, spend hours or years in therapy, often with no or little results. Only if you connect feeling and start working with feeling did clients really have a result. Focusing is a 6-step method that was developed from this understanding.

Another way to work with and change your feelings is to work with their qualities.

Let me invite you to a little experiment.

Make yourself comfortable then locate any feeling of nervousness, discomfort or strangeness within you.

Focus on where exactly you feel it: in your belly, your throat... Don't judge it; just observe it. It might come as asurprise, but feelings have a shape, a texture, a colour, and usually spin in one direction.

Have a look what colour, shape and consistency your feeling is and check out in which direction is it spinning (clockwise or anti clockwise).

Now take the feeling outside your body and place it in front of you. See its shape and colour; remember which way it has been spinning in your body.

Imagine you have a button that allows you to spin the feeling in the opposite direction and you can spin it faster, faster and faster than I can speak. Spin, spin, and spin it. Now have a good look... Yes, it should have changed its colour.

Once it has changed its colour take it back into your body, welcome it and start it moving and spinning in its new direction...

This can make a huge difference to how you feel. Any time the feeling wants to go back into its old direction, just remember the button and keep on spinning it in its new way. This works well to change negative feelings, but you can also use this for positive feelings: keep the direction and just let it spin faster and bigger and faster and bigger and let the good feelings radiate all through your body!

How to make yourself at home when you are not at home

Your limbic system is the gatekeeper to your senses. It is only fairly recently that it has been recognised for the complex system that it is, connecting our memories, our emotions and our sexuality. Understanding this gives you the opportunity to use sensory stimuli of all sorts — a favourite photo, a much-loved piece of music — to bring up positive memories and combat the feeling of being in a strange place.

There are many techniques to keep your limbic system happy and trigger feelings of relaxation and wellbeing. The following tips are tried and tested:

- Create a playlist of your favourite music and start listening to it every day while you practise your relaxation and breathing exercises.

- Hospitals have their own distinctive smell: you can block it out and boost your limbic system by putting a few drops of aroma oil on a tissue or burning it in a burner (if allowed). Oils or sprays work equally well, but make sure you use a natural aroma oil: rose, jasmine, ylang ylang – or whatever your nose likes best.

- Feel free to bring your own clothes: wearing a hospital gown is a strange experience and can make you feel exposed and uncomfortable. It should be something that you like to wear for relaxing at home and that will let you move around easily and take up whatever position you feel best in.

- Some women like to bring in their own pillow or a shawl.

- Find out what kind of lighting the hospital has and if it can't be dimmed, consider bringing in a battery-operated camping lantern, so that you can create soft lighting in the birthing room or round the birthing pool safely. (Most places will not let you use candles because oxygen is available in delivery rooms.)

- Imagine you are going away for the weekend and you want to make your hotel room a bit more home-like. Which photo or picture (it could even be a postcard) would you put up? Choose something that will keep you going and remind you of why you are here today.

Training your brain

A personal story

Throughout my life and my career as a midwife I have continued to research and to investigate different ways to make giving birth a better experience. In all the years since 1983, when I was a midwifery student, I have kept my eyes, ears, heart and mind open to learn to understand and support women giving birth, and it has been a long and interesting journey.

When I was thirty, I suffered very badly from migraines, and I consulted a doctor who used hypnosis. I was very keen to take part in a session, so he agreed to do a couple. To this day I can remember the difference between the sessions we did. The first was a pleasant trance in which we walked in beautiful surroundings, cleared some space and investigated a number of different areas, whereas in the second session I went in so deep that all I can remember is my conscious mind counting down and asking myself when the doctor was going to say something, then the next moment I woke up and to my amazement a whole hour had gone by. But I felt so good, so energised – I had not felt like that for a very long time, and what's more the feeling lasted for a very long time.

Hypnosis was not in fact very popular at that time, and it wasn't until many years later, when I went to New Zealand, that I came across it again, when I went to a talk on it. I then went to the United Kingdom to train in hypnosis, and I loved the results, and the feeling of getting in touch with 'my best friend on the other side'.

As I've said, everyone has a 'best friend on the other side' within themselves – your Dr Feelgood! This person has the extraordinary power to make you feel good, strong, relaxed and positive, and to keep you in this positive frame of mind. They are a real part of you, and through hypnosis you can feel, see and pay heed to this part of you more easily.

During my studies of hypnosis and neurolinguistic programming (NLP) in three different countries I have been intrigued by the way our minds create our thoughts, our beliefs, and our responses to all kinds of situations in daily life. I am even more amazed at how effectively the mind can control sensations in the body, even our perceptions of pain. If we can get in touch with this part of ourselves, we can let go of unwanted fears and thoughts, and create a positive and expansive self, ready to achieve the best possible birth.

 'Rain, after all, is only rain; it is not bad weather. So, also, pain is only pain, unless we resist it; then it becomes torment.'

The I Ching

Since 2005 have I worked with hundreds of mums who have used NLP successfully to get the birth they want. Give it a go: this has been around for a long time and is a fundamental part of releasing fears and traumas of all kinds.

It's useful to start the following exercises as early as you can, since the more relaxed you are throughout your pregnancy, the more positive the effect on your baby as well as on the birth. (Athletes often prepare themselves by using these methods. They visualise how they will run the race and see themselves crossing the finishing line as the winner.)

Paul McKenna says, 'The changes that matter most are often the changes in perception rather than changes in the world outside us.'

The fact is we can change the way we perceive the world and our image of pregnancy in a heartbeat.

If you don't take control of your birth, someone else will. It's as if you were a vegetarian and went to a restaurant, where you simply told the waiter that you were hungry and asked him to bring you some food. Now he might, with the best of intentions, bring you a juicy steak, which is his favourite food, and as far as he is concerned he has fulfilled your requirements completely. But is this really what you want?

Let's look into this method a bit more closely and find out how you can create a positive picture in your mind that will help you move more easily through the different stages of labour.

The power of imagination

This little exercise goes a long way to showing us how the mind works:

* Close your eyes and imagine yourself in your kitchen; look around and enjoy being in your kitchen.

* On the table there is a chopping board, and on the chopping board there is a beautiful lemon. It's a vivid yellow.

* Pick the lemon up, feel its weight, the texture of its skin, and notice its fresh smell.

* There's a knife next to the chopping board. Cut the lemon in half and see the juice running across the board. Smell the fresh smell.

✦ Now quickly pick up a piece, bring it up to your nose, and then take a big bite out of it — what a sensation in your mouth! Taste the fresh taste of the juice on your tongue.

Now open your eyes: there was no kitchen, no lemon, and yet you experienced all the sensations as if you had really cut into and eaten a lemon.

Now you know how to harness your imagination we are going to use it to create a positive picture of giving birth. But for this to be successful, you will need three things that you would need to achieve any goal:

1. You must want to achieve it.

2. You must know how to achieve it.

3. You must allow yourself to achieve it.

Redecorating

All our feelings come from the inside; they are an internal process even though we might display a reaction on the outside, perhaps in our breathing, our posture or our facial expressions. One way of changing the feelings on the inside is to stop and change the external reaction of the body, breathing deeply and calmly, straightening up your body and smiling.

'If you can dream it, you can do it.'
Walt Disney

So how can we change the images and feelings inside our bodies? Some time ago I went to a great workshop with Paul McKenna and Richard Bandler, the co-founder of neurolinguistic programming. Richard Bandler said something along the lines of, 'Suppose

I came round to your house and painted a horrible picture on y
wall. Wouldn't you redecorate straight away? And yet people go
around with horrible pictures inside them and never think to do
any internal redecorating; instead they carry on reliving their
fears.' Time to redecorate the chamber of horrors, I think.

Let's do this redecorating through a birth-oriented exercise that's
fun and works very well.

* Think of any anxieties you might have about childbirth, for
  example, that giving birth to a first baby will be long and
  painful; I won't be able to get the birth I want; I don't know
  if I will have the strength to go through labour; I might tear;
  all my friends had an epidural or a C-section.

* Focus on the image of that anxiety in your mind: is it a
  colour image or black and white? Are you visualising it in
  front of you, or to the right or the left? Is it a large image or
  a small image? A light image or a dark image? Is it a still
  photo or a moving image?

* If you're seeing a moving image, stop it and make it a still.

* If you're seeing this image in glorious Technicolor, let it fade
  to sepia.

* Let a black and white image become all blurry and lacking
  in contrast.

* If there is sound, turn it down so you can't hear it any more.

* Shrink the image so that it is so tiny you can tuck it under
  one fingernail, or move it so far away you can't make out
  what's in it anyway.

This technique works so well it could change your life forever.

Case study: developing a positive outlook

One woman in my care, let's call her Esther, used this technique very successfully. She came to me during her second pregnancy. During her first pregnancy she had read a bit about hypnosis, but had not consulted anyone about it.

When her labour took an unexpected turn and she ended up having to have a C-section, she was devastated. She came to see me second time around specifically so we could work together on her fears and the negative images that plagued her.

In a few sessions she had strengthened her positive outlook and also enhanced her ability to relax as she developed her skill in changing the pictures in her mind. When she finally gave birth to her beautiful baby she told me that using all those skills had made all the difference to her.

Pregnant or not, this is a great skill to have for the rest of your life!

Repainting reactions

It does us good to reach down into ourselves and release fears and negative emotions. Of course a degree of fear is healthy, and helps to keep us safe: standing back from the edge of a precipice is a good idea, but when fear comes to paralyse us in our choices, it can block positive action.

 'Start by doing what is necessary, then what is possible, and suddenly you are doing the impossible.'

Saint Francis of Assisi

The following exercise is designed to help you to let go of bad feelings and change your reactions or behaviours, especially if they don't seem to fit with your authentic, more positive self. It's an exercise that you can do as often as you want, and, like all the exercises in this book, you can use it for the rest of your life. So let's get right into it, because the sooner you start to anchor good feelings, the sooner it will become an automatic approach to life. And don't forget, just smiling helps too!

* Think of a reaction or behaviour you would like to change.

* Close your eyes and observe from your perspective what actually happens; try to identify the starting point of the reaction.

* Put a frame around this image and make it really vivid.

* Now observe yourself as if from the outside, displaying the desired reaction or behaviour. Notice how you act, hear what you say, and see what you see. Make sure this new reaction feels better to you than how you would have reacted previously.

* Shrink this perfect image into a small dark square and move to where you saw the first image.

* Now have the first image darken and shrink while you let the second picture become bigger and brighter until it completely obliterates the first picture. Imagine – or even make — a whooshing sound as this happens.

* Open your eyes.

Repeat this exercise three to five times, and then go back to the starting point of your original reaction. For most people it is very difficult to recapture the original feeling, as by now the new reaction seems to have supplanted the earlier one.

How to change the movie in your head

The two wolves

One evening an elderly Cherokee brave told his grandson about the battle that goes on inside people.

'My boy,' he said, 'The battle is between two 'wolves' who live inside all of us. One is evil; it is anger, envy, jealousy, sorrow, regret, greed, arrogance, self-pity, guilt, resentment, a sense of inferiority, lies, false pride, a sense of superiority, and ego.

'The other is good; it is joy, peace, love, hope, serenity, humility, kindness, benevolence, empathy, generosity, truth, compassion and faith. '

The grandson thought about this for a minute and then asked his grandfather, 'Which wolf wins?'

The old Cherokee simply replied, 'The one that you feed.'

I love this little story because it illustrates perfectly one of the most significant truths about our lives: our fate is in our hands. Even though we all carry these two wolves inside us, we have a choice as to which one we feed. The emotions we feed have a powerful influence on how we live our lives, and, as part of that, our experience of giving birth. We can keep on feeding our doubts and fears, or we can take a decision to feed our confidence, trust, and inner strength instead.

Stepping out of our comfort zone, feeling positive about something that we might be doing for the very first time – all of this is like a trip to a new country. To do this you need confidence and faith that, although it might look hard, you will be able to do it. The good news is – and I'm sure you'll agree with me –

when you feel happy, confident, and full of joy and willingness, things just happen more easily. I know you'll be able to adopt this approach if you feed the right wolf, so in the next exercise I'll show you how to let go of your fears and doubts, and feel confident about yourself, the upcoming birth, your baby, and the time after this amazing event. Life is too short to waste on fears and doubts: let go of them, feel more confident every day, and get the birth you really want – you deserve it!

What follows is a more extended exercise that follows naturally from the previous one. It's an effective exercise not only for the mother but for anyone involved in the birth, and it can really change your mind-set. Even if you don't think you have any particular anxieties, give it a try, as it also works with unconscious fears and doubts. Either tape the instructions, or ask someone to read them out to you softly and clearly. Make yourself comfortable, relax completely, and allow your eyes to close before you start.

* Lie down and allow yourself to relax completely.

* Be aware of the feel of the surface beneath you, the temperature of your hands... ... all of this is beginning to help you focus more closely on what is inside.

* Start inhaling love and good feelings down and around your baby in one line.

* Open your lips gently... exhale softly on a long breath out.

* Gently inhale love and relaxation down and once around your baby in one line.

* Gently exhale, letting go of any tension, any worries or negative thoughts.

✦ Keep on breathing softly and gently, and notice that the better you feel the more relaxed you are, and the more relaxed you are the better you feel.

✦ While you are breathing yourself into this beautiful state of deep relaxation, you and your baby are becoming so well connected, so safe, so secure...

✦ Imagine a drop of relaxation gently landing on the top of your head and starting to run down your body in all the colours of the rainbow.

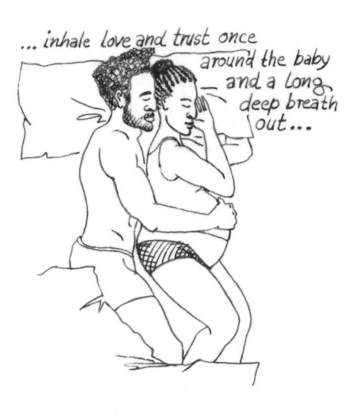

... inhale love and trust once around the baby and a long deep breath out...

* See all the colours of the rainbow all around you, while any tension just dissolves like snow melting in the spring sun and turning into a beautiful stream, a flow of clean fresh water.

* You could even form a small circle with your fingers and picture the circle of life and birth as your fingers touch...

* You can feel the relaxation running through your body like small, beautiful waves, from the top of your head down to the soles of your feet.

* It feels good to be so relaxed; relaxation really is a gift to yourself.

* And as you feel the waves of relaxation running through your body, allow waves of calm and peaceful feelings to flow from your head down your neck.

* It feels so good and so nice just to let go of any tension, any thoughts, any fears or worries.

* No one can disturb you; this is your time.

* While you wander through the landscape of your mind, any sounds from the inside or sounds from the outside will help you to relax even more deeply.

* Start to concentrate on the small muscles next to and around your eyelids, and start to relax the small muscles next to and around your eyelids. It might surprise you but the more relaxed those little muscles next to and around your eyelids are, the tighter your eyes are going to close...

* The tighter they close the more relaxed you are, the more

relaxed you are the deeper you, the deeper you go, the more you relax...

★ You know you could open them at any time, but why would you want to? It feels so good to relax so deeply and to teach your body this wonderful state of relaxation, the one you are going to reach during the birth as each contraction takes you deeper into relaxation, and the more relaxed you are... the gentler the birth will be.

★ Picture your favourite place in nature; it could be a place from the past, the present, or from your imagination.

★ Take a good look around and enjoy all the vibrant colours of nature. This is a place where you can be alone and never feel lonely...

★ ... a place so safe and so secure that you are going to leave your conscious mind here for a rest while you walk along with me. The ground is safe and secure beneath your feet.

★ Take a nice, deep breath and enjoy the freshness of nature. Look around and see the vibrant colours all around you. A gentle breeze touching your face feels good. You are part of the natural rhythm and nature is part of you.

★ Thoughts come and go, floating through the landscape of your mind, and you just let go. Enjoy letting go of worries, doubts and negative thoughts.

★ You can already feel how wonderful it is just to relax deeply and to realise who you really are.

★ Now you are ready to continue the journey into your inner wisdom... to the source of your inner wisdom.

* I am going to count down from ten to one, and while I am counting you will go further down into a deep and soothing relaxation.

* Ten: with each inhalation and exhalation letting go becomes easier and easier...

* Nine: you are going deeper into this inner space of love and harmony...

* Eight: gently further down, knowing that birth is a natural process...

* Seven: gently moving down feeling excited for all the things to come...

* Six: deeper and deeper into the inner peace of body wisdom, and the knowledge that the body that knows how to grow this baby also knows how to birth this baby...

* Five: getting closer to your inner connection, knowing that birth is as old as we are...

* Four: feeling happy and confident...

* Three: nearing the space where your mind and your body work together effortlessly...

* Two: reaching this space that is easy to trust, where you can learn how to bring your baby gently and effortlessly into the world...

* One: you are now in this special place of your own power, the power that you were born with, the power and strength to live a happy and fulfilled life.

✦ And as you let go, see yourself in your mind's eye, standing in front of a beautiful old door. As the door gently swings open, you enter a space within yourself – a room that everyone is born with: your place for resting, recharging your inner strength, for healing. The most beautiful room, shimmering in soft colours of blue, green, turquoise and a golden light

✦ Take a good look around you and notice a comfortable-looking armchair.

✦ As you make yourself comfortable in the armchair you can feel as the back of the chair supports you. Relax into the chair and just let go.

✦ As you look around you see a big book like an album and a pair of glasses lying on a table next to the armchair.

✦ It is a the most beautiful album, filled with stories, memories, pictures and photos of your life, experience, beliefs and opinions as recorded in the library of your inner self. The album contains your stories, stories that other people have told you, stories you found in the media, even stories from friends, family, books, movies, YouTube, Google...

✦ You put on the glasses to make sure that you can look at all those images free from strong emotion.

✦ Watch yourself sitting in the armchair, opening your album and flicking through the pictures and memories and stories of your life.

✦ Every time you find an image that triggers negative feelings, stop and realise what it really means for you: a bad experience that someone else had, as they were not as well prepared as you; the fear that you might not have the life you want; the fear that someone else will take control of your birth.

* Whatever the image is, look at it and make it bigger and bigger, then take all the colours out of it; make it fuzzier and lighter and fuzzier, until all the colours dissolve and it fades into the page until there is nothing left... just the beautiful structure of the paper.

* Then tear the page out of the book, scrunch it up and throw it into a basket right next to you.

* Your subconscious, your friend on the other side, is working fast, and keeps on going as you continue to flick through those memories and images.

* When you find the next negative one, see it for what it really is. Dissolve the image, the colours, letting it get bigger, fuzzier and paler, paler, paler, until all that is left dissolves into the page so that only the beautiful structure of the paper is left.

* Then tear the page out of the book, scrunch it up and throw it into a basket right next to you.

* Your subconscious is working fast as you flick through those pages.

* Whenever you come across an image that creates doubts, worries or fears about the upcoming birth or the time after, stop. Let it get fuzzier and fuzzier, paler and paler, let it go,

as the colour and the image dissolve right into the page – the page is like a sponge absorbing and erasing the image.

✸ All that is left is a beautiful empty page. Tear the page out of the book, scrunch it up and throw it into a basket right next to you.

✸ (Go through this exercise four to six times.)

✸ And now, finally, it is almost time to finish.

✸ See yourself in your mind's eye picking up the basket and pushing everything tightly down into it.

✸ As you stand up you realise there is a basin at the very back of the room. It is filled with a clear solution that allows you to see right down to the bottom of it.

✸ As you throw the scrunched-up paper into the basin, you can see the solution quickly dissolving the paper until only once again there is only a clear liquid left.

✸ You pull a huge lever and all the liquid quickly flows down the drain into the earth in a spiral motion and the vanished images are no longer part of your inner world.

✸ As the fluid disappears down the drain you feel so light, so happy and cheerful.

✸ You walk back to your chair, sit down and notice a screen right in front of you. The light dims and a movie starts playing.

✸ It's about you and your beautiful birth story.

✸ As the movie begins to play, you see yourself as your labour of love starts; you see yourself breathing through each and every contraction in a wave-like motion. As the picture moves, you see yourself moving in harmony with your body, your baby and your birth partner.

* And finally you see the image of you and your baby – WOW! The birth is over and you see yourself holding your baby skin to skin, your birthing partner next to you. The picture radiates love and happiness.

* You stop the movie here. This is the picture you want to keep: everything shimmers and shines in your favourite colours.

* Look at the picture and now make the colours brighter and more vivid; make the image bigger and bigger, and once it has reached life size, jump right into it.

* And now see what you see, hear the voices of your partner and the sweet sounds of your baby, and feel the feeling of success, feel the happiness, feel the weight of your baby's sweet body on your body.

* You have done it! And you have surprised even yourself – you had the birth you really wanted. Enjoy the feeling with each and every fibre of your body

* From now on, this is the picture that will come to into your mind every time you think about giving birth.

* This is the picture of your birth. Keep it, make it bigger, make it more colourful.

* Find the place of the good feeling inside yourself and start spinning it faster and faster. Let the good feeling move up and down your body until all you can feel is success, happiness and wellbeing.

✳ And now it is almost time to come back.

✳ Give yourself a moment to imagine that a fairy has flown into your home and touched you with her magic wand. What would be different?

✳ Allow yourself to feel different and decide what you are going to do to remind yourself to feed the right wolf.

✳ And I'm now going to count slowly from one to five:

✳ One: you're feeling light, and so positive.

✳ Two: you're as refreshed and energised as if you had had eight hours' sleep.

✳ Three: you know how to let go more easily.

✳ Four: feeling confident and trusting, take a deep breath, wriggle your fingers and wriggle your toes.

✳ Five: open your eyes, stretch as if you are waking up in bed after a good night's sleep – you're now fully awake, energised and feeling good.

I hope you enjoyed this fantastic exercise. There are a couple of things that it's useful to do immediately after it:

✳ If you feel like it, you could go back to the picture of your success and make this picture really big inside your head, then move towards creating smaller pictures of all the steps you have taken to make your big picture come true.

✳ You can write down some of these steps, if you feel like it.

✳ You can create a picture or a collage of what your dream birth looks like.

Whatever you choose to do, you must definitely remind yourself of this picture as often as possible and reconnect with the feeling. The more detailed the picture you create of the whole birth story unfolding, including the sounds, the people, the sensations and emotions, the better it is. The more specific the image you conjure up in your mind, the more positive and powerful the influence it has on you.

Fight the fear

Fear is not a great partner during pregnancy and childbirth: it causes the release of a lot of stress hormones, which do not help during pregnancy and birth.

Case study: an obsessive fear

One day Hannah rang me and told me she was thirteen weeks pregnant, but that she had lost a baby the previous year in the early weeks of pregnancy. As she was a medical doctor herself, she knew a lot about pregnancy and child-birth, but she was still driven to go to the emergency department once a week to check that her baby was still alive. Every time she went to the toilet she would check to see if there was blood on the toilet paper. I really felt for her: it all sounded very stressful, and far removed from the joy of pregnancy.

After a couple of sessions of hypnotherapy/NLP with me she was able to enjoy her pregnancy just like any other woman. We did some more sessions of NLP and hypnosis to prepare her for the birth, and she joined the yoga class, all of which helped her to have a good birth.

olden umbilical cord: relaxing to connect with your baby

Self-hypnosis and relaxation are fantastic tools to make use of at any time during your pregnancy, the birth, and afterwards. Relaxation is a genuine gift to yourself, and it is so much easier to achieve mental change and to feel really good when you are intensely relaxed.

The more you learn how to relax during pregnancy the easier it will be to achieve a deep relaxation while you are giving birth. But you could just practise it if you want to take a short nap, if you are having problems sleeping, or simply because it feels so good.

The five-time countdown relaxation method

Make yourself comfortable and allow yourself to fall asleep easily and effortlessly at any time during this session, give yourself permission to deeply relax:

* Now I am aware that I see the window

* Now I am aware that I see the wall

* Now I am aware that I see the pillow

* Now I am aware that I see my hand

* Now I am aware that I see... (whatever it is that you see)

Then say to yourself 'Now I am aware of what I hear' and allow both internal and external sounds to relax you deeper and deeper still:

* Now I am aware of hearing the sounds from the street

* Now I am aware of hearing the sound of the clock

✴ Now I am aware of hearing my own breath

✴ Now I am aware of hearing the sounds in my room

Then say to yourself, 'Now I am aware of what I feel':

✴ Now I am aware of the feeling of the pillow underneath my head

✴ Now I am aware of the feeling of my body resting on the mat

✴ Now I am aware of the feeling of the temperature of my hands

✴ Now I am aware of my baby moving

In the next round, see, hear and feel things three times instead of four times, and with each successive round reduce it once more, until you are down to one. If you make it to one, you can just start again, but it's most likely that you will just let go and enter a deep state of relaxation while moving through what your senses are experiencing. Just enjoy this wonderful feeling.

Moving deeper

As you relax, allow your eyelids to close gently.

✴ Observe your breath: inhale love and the good feelings; when you exhale, let go of all the stress, the negative thoughts, and any worries you may have.

✴ Nothing can disturb you you let yourself drift effortless, deeper and deeper into calmness and harmony. With each and every breath you allow yourself to just deeply glide into relaxation. The deeper you go the better you feel, the better you feel the deeper you go, It feels so good to let go and to relax.

* Let your mind relax here, taking a rest enjoying the natural surroundings. Enjoy the vivid colours you can see all around you; you have nature all around you: you are part of nature and nature is part of you.

* In this space it is so easy to let go of worries, stress and negative thoughts and become deeply relaxed, with your thoughts wide open.

* You feel so nurtured here that almost without noticing it, you will sense the relaxation running down from the top of your head to the soles of your feet and lapping like a gentle wave through your body.

* To take you down into an even deeper relaxation start to count down from 40 to 0, doubling your relaxation every time you pass the milestone of 30, 20, and 10. You will go down deeper, and deeper, 5, 4, 3, 2, 1, 0. This deep relaxation is a prize you can achieve.

Connecting with your baby

Now your body and mind are freed to learn, understand and go on a little journey.

* See yourself as you travel through time and space: see all the great people you have met and all the good things that have happened to you, and that are yet to happen as you float in a big boat down the river of your life. The river flows, sometimes serenely, with gentle waves, and sometimes more strongly, when the waves rock you gently from side to side.

* See yourself arriving at a beautiful shore, with the sun

warming your back. Now you are approaching a gate; as you stretch out your hand towards it, it swings open all by itself, letting you in to your magic garden.

*   In this garden the most beautiful fruit of all is growing. It may still be a seed in the ground, it may be a bud on a tree, or it may already be a ripe fruit ready to drop. You are in the magical garden of your womb.

*   If you want to, you can observe your little baby inside your womb, well-protected, loved and nurtured. You can see what your little baby is doing: is it sleeping or is it awake? Is it sucking its thumb, moving its little legs, or just having a nap?

*   Feel the connection between the two of you, as if you are joined by a golden umbilical cord, two hearts beating together in love, trust, and faith.

*   You smile at your baby and your baby smiles at you; you send love, trust and harmony towards the baby, and it returns those feelings to you along the cord that joins you.

*   As these emotions travel back and forth between you, you feel in close connection with your baby, and that feels good. You can come back to visit, and to enjoy that connection any time.

*   And now it is almost time to take your leave. Look around you, knowing that whenever you want to, you can, with every beat of your heart, be sending love, trust and harmony to your beautiful baby.

*   As you count from 1 to 5, return from this amazing journey:
    *   Feel the softness and gentleness of the moment
    *   Feel energised

* Feel the strength of the connection with your baby
* Feel refreshed and positive
* Open your eyes, stretch as if it were first thing in the morning, and feel spiritually alive.

Summary

Chapter 3 has been all about how to tame your mind and train it to keep you positive – a great skill for life, not only for pregnancy and childbirth.

You have learnt to let go of unwanted fears, to swap the negative movie playing in your head for a joyful, optimistic one and to create a vibe around yourself that will keep you calm, relaxed and in control wherever you give birth.

By now you will have gathered that all the things you have learnt in this book are connected, each feeding into the other, and all of them working together to support you and your baby on this momentous occasion.

Goodbye... and thank you

As I finish writing this book in India, a cow has silently given birth to a little calf on the paddy field in front of my house. Life resonates with what goes on...

First of all, thanks to all the mothers, fathers, women – and babies – in the world that have never stopped asking me things and telling me to write this book. When I began writing it, like you, I had no idea what sort of journey I was on. As with pregnancy, birth and parenthood, writing – and indeed living – each brings its own surprises.

Many things have happened, and sometimes it feels as if the whole world is lacking in passion, oxytocin, peace, love happiness, and bonding. But giving birth carries a hidden magic: it teaches you trust, love and surrender. Passion and love together can unleash our hidden powers. We release oxytocin when we are making love as well as when we give birth, which helps us to connect at the deepest level. Giving birth can become the biggest resource in your life: a valuable bank of memories that you will be able to draw on for the rest of your life.

One woman said to me, 'Birth is the only blind date in your life that guarantees you will fall deeply in love.' How true! And this is how it should be. At a time when interventions in the process of birth have reached their highest level, it is vital that you prepare yourself well to ask questions and stand up for your rights, but on the other hand be ready to surrender and let go.

In spite of what is happening both in the wider world and in the world of childbirth, I remain an optimist. My mother would say I am a born optimist. We now know so much about the birthing process, the unborn baby, the newborn baby, attachment parenting, and yet intervention in birth is still on the rise. We are having to relearn the importance of bacteria and seeding, and to learn how to surrender, and trust our bodies and instincts. As an expectant mother, you have to be brave and ask the right questions. This is your journey, and you deserve the best experience in discovering the magic of birth. I guess I will always be an optimist, because I believe in our human capacity to learn and to change.

As we've moved from hormones to the body and the brain, I've shared with you both knowledge and the techniques I use myself in daily life: hypnosis, NLP, exercises. I enjoy doing this so much that I speak about it at conferences and share my knowledge not only with parents-to-be, but with other professionals in Germany, in Australia and, via Skype, all over the world.

I share with you my stories, my beliefs and my experiences because I want you to have a unique experience. Having a great birth is a wonderful experience for everyone involved, even the midwife, the doula, the doctor and the friends and family. So if you've liked my book, start sharing it with your friends and your community, and let me know how it goes. I'd love to hear your story, so send me an email and share your experience with me.

With the aim pf providing good childbirth education and fun-to-learn classes, I offer you my online programme www.elementsofbirth.com. This book is the childbirth strand within this platform, and I would love to welcome you to the website. There I can share my knowledge with you in your own time and as often as you like.

From small things big things grow, whether it is seeds in the ground, babies, or, as I truly believe, the future of our children, our society and our world. We hold these in our hands and we have to focus on them with more love. So join me on Facebook, YouTube, my programme or in a Skype session. I wish you a fearless, safe and happy birth.

Finally, here is a little exercise that you can do, maybe later today, or tonight, or maybe tomorrow:

Your subconscious is going to create a possibility, something 'wow!', to surprise you.

It is a present, like a gift, a very special gift, something exceptional, so beautiful: a wonderful feeling. It might come in a brilliant colour, a soothing sound, maybe even a delicious taste. It is something that stands out, a brilliant sensation of feeling good, perhaps only for a fleeting moment. It could be like a glimpse into the future, or a moment of bliss, or maybe an extended feeling of trust and wellbeing, a feeling that you are OK.

* It could be something like laughter or a rich feeling of inner wealth.

* It could be anything.

* Be aware of your subconscious, your best friend on the other side, and open your mind to beautiful things: feelings, experiences and moments.

* These special feelings will surprise you from now on, and you can enjoy them to the full.

Much love,
Jutta

Appendices

Appendix I: Creating your birth plan

The birth of your baby is a life-changing event, and hopefully it will be one of the happiest moments you will ever experience. In the weeks and months before the birth, you will want to spend time thinking through your hopes and desires for this magical moment. Creating a mind-map, writing a journal, drawing or painting, or using a diary will help you to list your priorities and wishes. Out of these you will be able to create a birth scenario that reflects your personal needs and wishes and distil this into a birth plan.

Birth plans have become more and more popular over the past few years. These days women have a clear vision of the sort of birth they want, yet hospitals are often understaffed and very busy. This is why it's very important to make sure people know and understand what you really want, and this can be quite a communication challenge.

A birth plan is usually a straightforward one-page statement, written in positive language, to let those where you will be giving birth know how you would like to be supported during the birth. It's a good idea to make a few copies of your birth plan available so that everyone who will be involved has a chance to read it through and discuss any issues with you well in advance of your due date.

Tip
Find out about your hospital: the most common intervention is induction of labour, but statistics show that every second woman induced will go for an epidural, and every second one of these

Much of the content of your birth plan will depend on where you are planning to give birth. If you are planning to give birth in a birthing centre, you may not need a very lengthy plan as these places are woman-centred and support natural childbirth. If you are planning to give birth in a hospital you should give them your birth plan quite some time before the big day so that all the doctors, midwives and other staff who might be involved in the birth have a chance to read it.

What do *you* want?

There are many aspects of the birth to be considered. You should have a clear picture of what you want, and once you know what it is, it will be easier to communicate it with others. But a good birth plan will not be rigid: a good birth plan should also allow you the opportunity to discuss important details with those who are caring for you. Bear in mind that sometimes things do not work out according to plan and leave room for manoeuvre in case special circumstances arise. A good birth plan should help you to achieve your goal, whatever happens.

Your health care providers

You need to find out what the standard routines and procedures are for expectant mothers. Most health care providers have guidelines and set procedures for the way they work. These are aimed at getting the best outcome for you and your baby, but it can mean that there is little flexibility. Some providers will be open to your wishes, but others might see your list as very demanding, or even as increasing certain risks.

Tip
Demand the best: you can only give birth to this baby once – this is not a holiday destination that you can revisit.

If you disagree with any of the procedures, or don't like them, you should discuss this with your health care provider, and in extreme cases you might need to change your provider – but this should be only if the worst comes to the worst. You should also discuss your thoughts with your birthing partner, so that they will be aware of them and be able to support you when the time comes.

The more you find out about what to expect, the more detail you'll be able to put into your plan. You can divide your birth plan into different sections, creating one page for a straightforward birth without any complications, and one to be used if special circumstances arrive.

The table below will help you to consider all aspects of the birth, from the professional care where you will be giving birth, to the domestic arrangements you may want to make the around the event itself. Just leave out anything that doesn't resonate with you.

Issues to consider	Options
How mobile do you want to be during labour, and what equipment do you want?	What kind of movement do you have in mind: walking/standing/squatting/kneeling/leaning? Will you need a tub, a ball, a rope?
	How about resting? You might want a mat, a pillow, a beanbag.
	What birthing positions might you want to adopt? A water birth, a birthing stool.
	Will you be able to go for a slow birth to avoid an episiotomy (which should only be done in exceptional circumstances)?
What kind of pain relief do you want?	Massage, hot packs, Tens machine, acupuncture, homeopathy, hypnosis, relaxation techniques, bathing, breathing, medication (should they offer this to you or will it be up to you to ask for it?).
What are foetal monitoring is a likely to be used and how do you feel about these methods?	A handheld Doppler machine, a pinnard (similar to a stethoscope), cardiotopograph, a machine for monitoring the baby's heartbeat
What about special circumstances?Can you do skin to skin straight away? Is there a chance for seeding in case of a C section ß	For births at home or in birthing centres, what are the arrangements for emergency transport in the case of an emergency?Have you any special requests if a Caesarean section is needed?

Issues to consider	Options
Who do you want to be present at the birth? It may depend on which country you are in as to how many people can be at the birth.	It could be your midwife with visiting rights to deliver your baby in the hospital, a doula, just the standard hospital team, your mother? Will there be any children/siblings of the baby present? If so, who will be tasked with looking after them? Do you offer full rooming-in or a family room?
How about eating and drinking during labour?	Do you want an IV line? (How to avoid it) How will you keep yourself hydrated? Will you want ice chips to suck?
What else will I be able to do to make myself feel comfortable?	Can I wear my own clothing? Can I bring my own music? Is the lighting in the room where'll be giving birth adjustable?
What will happen after the birth?	Will I be able to have skin-to-skin contact with my baby straight after the birth? Will I be able to have a lotus birth if I want to? Can I have the cord-clamping delayed? What do I need if I feel well enough to go home after the birth?

Writing your plan

Once you've decided on the content of your plan, it's important to set it down in a positive way. Partners and professionals will enjoy discussing it a lot more if it's not a long list of 'I don't want this, I don't want that'. Your birth plan will be much more appealing if it's expressed in terms of 'we hope to... ', we plan to... ', or 'we have prepared... ', as it will keep others more open to your wishes.

Your plan should let others know that you have been preparing yourself for the birth, and that you are looking forward to having them support you. Get them as excited as you are, and share your trust and confidence with them.

Here are a couple of examples of how you might phrase your wishes:

- As regards pain management, I have informed myself about all the options on offer, I understand what is available here, and would like to ask for them myself if I feel I need them.

- I would like to be able to move freely, and change position as often as I need to.

- It would be wonderful if I could use the bath tub as often as I like.

You could also create a list to cover any concerns you might have should an emergency arise, with questions such as 'Will my partner be able to stay with me? Will I be able to have skin-to-skin contact with my baby soon after the delivery? Will there be support for breastfeeding? Is seeding an option with a C section?

Using your birth plan

A birth plan will help you to keep your focus on the outcome you want, and give you confidence to express your wishes as you will be clear about what they are. If you've discussed your birth plan with your carer, you will have developed an understanding and will be speaking the same language on the day.

Bear in mind that during the birth, you and your birthing partner can ask for more information at any time and, unless you are in an emergency situation, ask for more time to make a decision.

Remember, birth is a natural process, and most women will have a normal birth. You can only give birth to this baby once, so be prepared to speak up for your wishes and dreams, and ask people to support you through this momentous event.

I wish you a Happy Birthing Day!

Appendix II: Special circumstances: How to use your skills whatever happens

This is a section for when women may find themselves in special circumstances. Some of you might need, for one reason or another, to have a C-section or some other sort of assistance for your baby. Even if a C-section is planned, you will still be able to use the information in this book to help you.

Applying the birth breathing will calm you and your baby before you go off to the operating theatre. If you can stay relaxed and happy, and breathe love and oxygen down to your baby, it will feel better and so will you. If you feel nervous and anxious at any time during your pregnancy and need to calm yourself down, it's great to breathe yourself into relaxation and focus on making the negative pictures in your mind smaller.

Tip
Whatever special circumstances apply in your case, ask to be informed about all the possible options.

Of course, if there are unmistakeable problems you will want to consult your midwife or another practitioner, but even in this situation keeping your mind free of fears and staying positive are the most helpful things you can do.

 'Nothing in life is to be feared. It is only to be understood.'
Marie Curie

Bear in mind that the 'fight or flight' mechanism is not designed to support the uterus, so to ensure your baby is well supplied with oxygen in a crisis you will need to focus on breathing and on remaining calm. Staying in touch with your baby in this way is the best thing you can do; your midwife, and maybe a doctor, will take care of all the rest.

Case study: tangled in the umbilical cord

When I first met Pia, pregnant with her first child, she was sitting in the bath, with labour well established. As I listened to the baby's heart, I could hear significant drops in the baby's heart rate, and only a slow recovery to a more acceptable level. I asked Pia to change her position in the bath, and to breathe deeply down and around her baby.

I listened in with each contraction, but I could tell that things were getting worse, not improving, so I asked Pia if I could examine her, to understand what was happening better. Unfortunately her cervix was only four centimetres dilated, and I could hear that the baby was getting very distressed, no matter what we did.

I decided to transfer Pia to the labour ward, and warned her and her partner that it was likely she that she would have to have a C-section. While everyone around us got busy, I practised birth breathing with Pia. What was amazing was that, although the baby's heart rate did not recover fully after each drop (contraction?), there was nevertheless a significant change. The midwifery student working alongside me that day also noticed the difference in the heart rate when Pia and I were breathing together.

There really was no option but a C-section: out came a tiny little girl wrapped up in the cord like a parcel. There was no way that she could have untangled herself to be born through the birth canal. Even so, Pia and her partner have good memories of the birth, during which they stayed calm, confident that they were actively supporting the baby in the best way they could. Needless to say, mother and baby had a long period of skin to skin contact and breastfeeding so that they could connect with each other and fall in love.

Case study: Ventouse extraction and how to use your skills

Flora had a healthy pregnancy, and was well prepared for the birth, having practised yoga and received acupuncture and 'Happy Birth Day' hypnosis.

Finally, ten days past her due date, she went into labour spontaneously. All went well at the hospital she had chosen, though the labour went on for a long time. Flora turned down the epidural the midwife offered her.

Flora and her partner were a good team, and the baby seemed to be doing well. After 15 hours, she was ready for the final stage, but her little girl had got stuck in the birth canal. Flora tried all the techniques she knew, but the baby's heart rate began to drop quite markedly. Her daughter was going to need help to be born and was eventually delivered via a Ventouse extraction (where a suction cup is attached to the baby's head to help pull the baby from the birth canal). The baby came into the world pink and alert, with a big cry, and was out straight onto her mother's chest.

Flora told me that even though it hadn't been quite the birth she had imagined, she still felt satisfied and empowered. She had used all her skills in relaxation, birth breathing, and in moving to find the best position while her daughter was being born, and she never felt a failure because she had been with her baby every step of the way. And that's what this process is all about.

Sometimes babies just get stuck and can't find their way out. Look on it as if you had gone hiking or climbing, and someone had given you a helping hand over the last few metres so you could finally enjoy the view.

Case study: C-section

Nina wanted to have a baby and for all sorts of reasons had difficulty conceiving. After an assisted conception, at the age of nearly 40, she became pregnant with twins. At first she was in shock, but then she realised that it was in fact a stroke of luck, as she wouldn't have to try all over again to get pregnant a second time.

Nina researched her options well and decided early on that she wanted me to be her midwife. The pregnancy was going well: she was super-healthy, working, cycling, enjoying yoga, and she never looked as though she was carrying twins.

But at one of her antenatal visits the scan showed that one of the babies had begun to grow more slowly, as sometimes happens with a twin pregnancy. Over the next couple of weeks it became clear that this baby was growing too slowly, and a decision was taken that she would have to have a C-section to deliver the babies. Nora was happy to have taken this decision, even though she had prepared for a natural birth, so we spent some time discussing how she could apply everything that she had learnt, to make sure that she would still have a great experience and be able to connect with her babies and breastfeed them.

She discussed her wishes with the delivery team and was able to have skin to skin contact with the babies when they were still in the operating theatre. She breastfed them as soon as they left the theatre. She later told me that she and her partner had a family room and spent their first days with the twins almost nude, cuddling, kissing and warming them.

This worked so well that when they were discharged on the sixth day the babies were already gaining weight well. At six months they were still breastfeeding. Nora told me that everything she had learnt was helpful during the pregnancy, enabled her to stay calm on the way into the theatre, and continued to be useful.

Case study: Big baby

Women are often told that they are carrying big babies, and that they should therefore have a C-section. Sometimes this is right, but sometimes nature can surprise us. Let me tell you the story of the biggest baby I have ever delivered.

One day I was on duty at the birthing centre when a woman pregnant with her second baby came in with well-established contractions. All was going well and she seemed very calm. I offered her a room and started filling a bath. She and her partner took their places in the bath and I went in every so often to check on the baby and offer my support.

After an hour or so, the woman started to change the sounds she was making, which was a sign to me that she might be ready to give birth. From her paperwork I had seen that her first baby had weighed over four kilos, and had only been delivered after a long labour involving an epidural and a drip, and finally a Ventouse extraction when the shoulders got stuck – all in all a very traumatic experience. I kept all this information in mind.

I supported when she started pushing, but after an hour I felt she was getting nowhere. She started crying, and saying that it would be just like last time. When I examined her, her cervix was fully dilated and the head seemed to be in a good position, so I wondered what was going on. After another hour with little progress, I rang a colleague to come and help me, just in case we were going to have trouble with the shoulders again. I suspected a pretty big baby was on its way.

Finally the head crowned, but when nothing had happened after a further hour, she demanded that I do an episiotomy. I refused, telling her that I did not do episiotomies unless it was absolutely necessary. She insisted, telling me she was sure the baby would come out if I did. I gave in and made a small incision. Sure enough the baby came out with the next contraction: the crown, the head, big chubby cheeks, and, before I could even think, his whole body slipped into the world: a huge, healthy boy, pink and crying out to go straight into his mother's arms.

I weighed him three times to be sure of what I was seeing: 5250 grammes and 60cm long. He was the star of the postnatal ward. His mother taught me that size doesn't have to dictate everything, and that sometimes miracles happen before your very eyes.

Appendix III: Your packing list

First of all, find out exactly what will be supplied by the hospital or birthing centre (for example, nappies). Then you might want to add the following things to the list that your birthing place will give you.

You

Clothes

* Your favourite top: it should be something you feel really comfortable in and that you have already been wearing for a while, as it will be a connection with home.

* A vest: for if you don't want to be naked in the bath. If you don't mind being naked in the bath, don't bother.

* Several items of your pregnancy underwear.

* Socks: sometimes when we're nervous our feet get cold, so you want to make sure that they are nice and warm, even though your body is going to heat up during the birth.

* Comfortable tops/tunics to wear after the birth; they should open easily at the front for breastfeeding. It's a good idea to go for something long enough for you to feel confident walking around in, but bear in mind that you will need to change pads (both breast pads and sanitary pads) frequently.

Food and drink

* Lollies to suck on, to moisten your lips.

* Some dextrose tablets to keep your energy up.

* Delicious snacks to have after the birth

Creature comforts

✳ A plastic bottle or a plastic cup with a straw: you need to drink while in labour, but you don- t want to have to worry about glass breaking.

✳ A pillow or shawl that smells of home can be helpful.

✳ A picture or small object that is dear to you, to remind you of why you are here.

✳ Your favourite aromatherapy oils (while you are pregnant that is!): rose or jasmine are very suitable, or it could even be plain almond oil. Make sure they are one hundred per cent natural, in case you get into a bath or birthing pool after your massage – you don- t want your baby born into any chemicals, or even into anything very strong like pepper-mint oil.

✳ If you are having a water birth, ask if they supply neck pillows, and if not, bring a small inflatable one of your own.

✳ Suitable lighting: although candles are not allowed for safety reasons, you could bring a battery lamp or a camping lantern to give off a soft and soothing light.

✳ Music: put together a playlist for your breathing and relax-ation exercises, as well as your favourite tracks, and bring something to play it on.

✳ Your camera and a charger or spare battery. It- s amazing to have some pictures from immediately after the birth (or even during the birth).

Your partner

✣ A copy of your birth plan.

✣ A prompt sheet for the birth breathing (see p. ¢).

✣ Sustaining snacks for and drinks for your partner during the birth – as they will be supporting you they won't have the opportunity to go off and have a meal!

✣ Two sets of comfortable clothes in their bag at all times, just in case they are summoned directly from work.

✣ A pair of swimming trunks in case he wants to get in the bath with you (sorry, but a naked man in a hospital or birthing centre is not that great!), or a swimsuit if your partner is your mother, sister or other female.

✣ A phone, charger, and the numbers of everyone they will want to call.

✣ With a second or subsequent child, a little present from the newborn for its sibling(s).

Appendix IV: Tips and tricks

Birth: the practicalities

✳ Prepare yourself; don't leave things till the last minute. Find a good class or join my online programme.

✳ Find a good place to give birth early in the pregnancy, visiting possible places (definitely check out a birth centre) and exploring all the issues like intervention rates, till you find a place you're really comfortable with.

✳ If home birth is available where you live, speak to a home birth midwife.

✳ If you are having a planned C-section, talk to your midwife about how you can best prepare for this. Check out 'seeding' a new method aimed at making sure the baby can still benefit from the mother's good bacteria, and find out what you can do to catch up with your hormones.

✳ Put up a sign outside wherever you are giving birth that reads 'Shhh, birth in progress. Please respect this and be quiet!'

✳ Get your birthing bag ready at around thirty-seven weeks; having everything ready will keep your stress levels down.

✳ Empty your bladder often during giving birth: a full bladder can stall the birth and make it difficult for the baby's head to go down the birth canal.

✳ If what you're doing doesn't work, don't do more of the same; try doing the opposite.

Food and drink

* Get plenty of iron by eating oats, lentils, broccoli, egg yolks, and red grapes. All dark green and dark red foods, and sugar beet molasses, will keep your iron levels up.

* Eat fresh and healthy foods at least five times a day in pregnancy, as your metabolism changes.

* Linseed and chia seeds will maintain your omega-3 and omega-6 levels, as will even small amounts of ocean fish.

* Keep lots of healthy snacks in your bag, such as nuts, seeds and dried fruit. Dried apricots are a great source of calcium and magnesium.

* Eating an avocado a day will give you healthy amino acids. (Fish and meat also contain amino acids.)

* Drink lots of water during the pregnancy and while you are giving birth to stay well-hydrated. Going without just one glass of water makes your brain slow down, causing you to feel low, tired, and unmotivated.

* Start drinking a birth tea from 36 weeks onwards: it should be a mixture of lady's mantle and horsetail to strengthen the uterus and increase your iron levels, and raspberry leaf to prepare the cervix. Take one or two cups a day.

* A study published in the *Journal of Obstetrics and Gynaecology* concluded that eating six dates daily during the last four weeks of pregnancy 'significantly reduced the need for induction and augmentation of labour, and produced a more favourable... delivery outcome.'

* Go as vegetarian as you can in the last weeks of your

pregnancy. These days most people are hyperacidic, and this can result in more pain in your muscles and joints. Eating lots of fresh fruit and vegetables and drinking water (preferably warm) creates a good basic environment in your body.

* If you suffer from swollen feet, legs and hands, eat cooked potatoes, fresh pineapple, asparagus, together with protein from eggs or cottage cheese, and drink lots of water. If that doesn't help, try acupuncture. (This is assuming your blood pressure and blood analyses are normal.)

* If you are constipated, try raspberries – even frozen ones will work – or other berries. They are a great source of roughage.

* When you prepare nice food, make some extra portions to stick in the freezer, ready for after the birth.

Looking after your body

* Go for a long walk every day. It will help your legs and back to feel better.

* Start massaging your perineum from thirty-six weeks onwards if it feels right to you. (Maybe your partner would like to be involved.) A study has shown that this can help to prevent tears.

* Getting acupuncture from thirty-six weeks onwards is a great way to prepare for the birth.

* Practise this easy pelvic floor exercise: imagine you have your favourite drink underneath you, and you're holding a straw in your vagina. Inhale, making a slurping noise and

picturing yourself sucking the drink up, and hold for a count of five, then release. Do this whenever you see the colour red or green – just do it!

* Do your birth breathing every day – practice makes perfect.

* Practise yoga, Qi Gong, Tai Chi or meditation during your pregnancy: they help you learn to relax and provide additional resources that you can use on the day.

* Go swimming – it's great to experience buoyancy during pregnancy.

* Bathe in Epsom salts or in the sea: both are great ways to detoxify and cleanse the body.

* If your blood pressure is low drink lots of water and use rosemary oil, perhaps in a bath, as it helps blood pressure to go up.

* If you like beauty treatments, have waxing and a manicure and pedicure before the birth – it may be a while before you feel comfortable having these things done again.

* Use natural products on your skin and deodorants without aluminium: chemicals are absorbed into your body through your skin, hair and nails, and you won't want your baby exposed to them.

Accentuate the positive

* Create a mind map for your birth: paint, write, draw pictures, glue photos – whatever you want.

* Have a clear idea in your mind about the birth you want. Studies have shown that those who write down their goals

in life, or their new year resolutions, were more successful in achieving them. Giving birth is not a goal-oriented activity but this is still good mental preparation and a good way to connect with your baby.

* Visualise your cervix opening and the baby slipping through.

* Never listen to bad birth stories; plug your ears, smile, and say 'I will listen to this six months after the birth of my baby.'

* If you can't sleep, stop negative thoughts by exercising and taking a warm bath with lavender.

* Join a pregnancy yoga group to meet like-minded mums. Yoga is an excellent way to prepare yourself both physically, through breathing and movement, and mentally for the birth. That,s why I love it and teach it.

* Do the fear release exercise as often as you need to.

* Take time to get in touch with your baby, massaging your belly frequently, and humming or singing.

* From the very first moment that you are aware you are pregnant until you hold the baby in your arms, visualise it and focus on your feelings towards it: this really will create a change in your brain.

* Human beings have the unique ability to create their reality internally and then superimpose it on the outside world. Make use of that by changing the movie in your head into a joyful birthing movie.

* Using positive language during the birth will support you through the process.

You and your partner

✳ Enjoy your last weeks alone with your partner: do something special like having a romantic candle-lit dinner.

✳ A woman has four hands after the birth: two belong to her and two belong to her partner.

✳ Do a 'dry run' with your partner: set your alarm to go off every three hours (you might be breastfeeding as often as this), and each time discuss who is going to do what.

Appendix V: Birth breathing prompt sheet

Photocopy or take a photo of this page so you can have it by your side during the birth, and make sure your birthing partner knows it's there.

Keep everything soft: your shoulders, face, lips are all soft and relaxed.

1. Inhale through your nose...
2. ... down in one line...
3. ... once, love around the baby ...
4. ... and a long deep breath out (SSSSHHHHhhhh).

1. A soft breath in...
2. ... down in one line...
3. ... love once around your baby...
4. ... and a long deep breath out.

1. A gentle breath in...
2. ... down in one line...
3. ... love once around your baby...
4. ... and a l-o-o-o-o-n-g deep breath out (lips open: everything comes out while you're breathing out).

Now the contraction is finished: breathe normally, lips, soft, cheeks soft, shoulders soft – all of your body is so soft and so relaxed.

And so on.

When you feel like it, take a break: move, kiss, eat, drink, relax, change your position.

A little tip: you don't have to keep on using the words, just breathe together, focusing on happy images and feelings about your baby.

Appendix VI: Frequently asked questions

When will I first feel my baby's movements?

If you are pregnant with your first baby, you could start to feel something at eighteen weeks, or it could take until twenty-two weeks. It might be hard to recognise to begin with: it feels a bit like the flutter of butterfly wings, or as if you had a fish swimming around in you! When the baby is bigger, you will definitely feel it kicking.

Is it ok to make love during the pregnancy? My partner is afraid of hurting the baby.

If you have a healthy pregnancy and you feel like making love, it's absolutely fine. If you feel good, your baby feels good, and what helped it in helps it out as well!

Can I, or should I, exercise during my pregnancy?

Yes, yes, and yes again! And you can choose from a great variety of exercise. Go for something you enjoy, and that offers strength, alignment, and some relaxation. Don't do too much running or jumping, out of consideration for your pelvic floor.

I have been teaching pregnancy yoga for many years, and I love the connection it makes between the body, the mind, breath and movement.

Join a class, or get a DVD if you live too far away. Pregnancy classes have the advantage of putting you in touch with other women, and it's fun to see bellies of all shapes and sizes from six to forty-two weeks! Try to find an experienced instructor who will be able to adapt their class to any particular needs you might have.

I've been invited to a social event where most people will be drinking. Is it OK to have a small one?

NO – absolutely not! I have a zero alcohol policy. Research from some years back established through ultrasound that even after a small amount of alcohol babies were in effect drunk in the womb. Their livers are unable to process alcohol. If you love your baby, just ask for water or juice.

Is it safe to fly during pregnancy?

Yes, it is, but always check with the airline up to what date they will take you. If you will be flying for longer than ten hours, you need to be aware that you could develop a blood clot. That's why you must drink lots of water, wear compression stockings, exercise your feet and legs during the flight, and get up and wander around as much as possible. Fasten the seat belt under your belly. You could also try a homeopathic remedy: Lachesis d6/d12/ or c6, 3–5 globules, three to four times a day. Bon voyage!

Home birth, birth centre, hospital? Where should I go?

To be honest, it will depend a lot on where you live, what's available and so on. Although I'm a big fan of home births and birthing centres, I have worked in hospitals as well, and let's face it, most women do give birth in hospitals. My advice to you is to get as much information as possible about what would be available for you and keep your options open. Even if you think a home birth or a birthing centre might not be for you, speak to your midwife, visit a birthing centre, and find out all about it. Then decide on what **you** feel happiest with – not what your friends or your doctor would prefer. If you leave it until the last moment, you won't even get a chance to choose.

Even within Europe, there are huge differences from country to country: in Germany, you have a free choice of where to give birth. In Australia, though, where you go will depend to a large extent on your postcode.

Outcomes for birthing centres are very good, with low levels of intervention and, of course, a hugely supportive environment. Research has established that for a low-risk pregnancy a home birth with a professional midwife is safe. The reasons for the low uptake of home births and birthing centres are political as much as anything: I recommend a viewing of *The Business of Being Born*.

If you decide on a hospital, discuss your birth plan with them, and explore whether they would allow a midwife with visiting rights to attend you.

Above all, choose your midwife carefully: they are the experts on a normal pregnancy, birth, and the time after. You'll want to establish a good relationship with her: Thirty-eight to forty-two weeks is a long time!

What should I do if I need a C-section?
Even if you'll be having a planned C-section, you should still have a birth plan ready. You'll be able to use many of the skills, like the breathing and massage techniques, before you get to the theatre, and the hypno-birthing mind exercises will help you to stay calm during the whole procedure and to handle the pain and discomfort you might experience in the first days.

You should ask to have skin-to-skin contact in the baby while still in the theatre, and if for any reason you yourself cannot do this, your birthing partner should be able to have skin-to-skin contact with the baby, speak to it, etc.

If you can, spend the next few days in a family room, kissing and cuddling the baby, and feeding it as much as you can.

The latest studies have shown that babies born through C-sections miss out on exposure to a lot of good bacteria, so some women opt for 'seeding': you swab your vagina and then wipe the baby's nose and mouth with the swab, so that it comes into contact with your bacteria.

I'd also advise going to see a chiropractor or an osteopath after the birth, so that they can release some of the tension from the baby's head. You can get some insights into this practice by watching the film *Microbirth.*

My appetite is on the increase. Is it true that I have to eat for two?

This is not quite true. Once you are past the first few weeks, you might suddenly experience cravings for the strangest things, and you can follow the dictates of your body to a degree, but there's no need literally to eat for two. The baby will take whatever it needs from what you eat. Just have a good healthy diet, and note whether any cravings you may experience are because your blood sugar is low. Carry healthy snacks with you, like nuts, dried apricots and apples. You're better off having five small meals a day than two or three really big ones.

My partner doesn't want to come to the birth – he is too afraid.

First of all, have him read this book, ask him what he is afraid of, and take him to a really good ante-natal class. (He could also do my on-line programme with you.) If he still doesn't want to come to the birth, you have to accept his decision. It won't help to have someone full of fear with you at the birth.

Find someone you trust to come and support you. You could even look for a doula – a woman who specialises in providing birth support. Some are very good and will perform all the tasks you would expect a birthing partner to perform, such as rubbing your back, running a bath, etc. (Doulas are more common in countries where there are few midwives.) They can be wonderful, but again, you need to choose carefully and, of course, be able to pay to engage one.

Is it OK to stay on a vegetarian or even a vegan diet during the pregnancy?
In general, yes, but only if you know a reasonable amount about nutrition. You will have to make sure you get enough vitamins, protein, and omega 3 and 6. It will take a bit more effort, and you might have to watch your weight. Introduce chia seeds, linseed, tofu, nuts and pulses into your daily diet, and make sure it is well-balanced overall. You might want to take a kelp supplement.

Further resources

My Elements of Birth resources

Happy Birthing Days online course

Elements of Birth yoga DVD (below), online community, YouTube channel and live webinars.

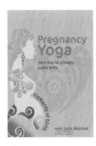

See my website http://elementsofbirth.com/ for more information on all of these.

Books and downloads

Balaskas, J. (1990). *New Active Birth: A Concise Guide to Natural Childbirth.* **London: Thorsons. (Kindle edition available.)**
Although it's an older book, this is still a great read. Janet Balaskas is a midwife who used to run a water birth practice in London, and her book is full of practical advice.

Bandler, R. & McKenna, P. (2008). *Get the Life You Want.* **London: Harper Element.**
This book teaches you great techniques from neuro-linguistic programming (NLP) for achieving whatever you want to achieve. Of course I love it; I'm an NLP trainer!

Buckley, S. J. (2009). *Gentle Birth, Gentle Mothering: A doctor's guide to natural childbirth and gentle early parenting options.* **Berkeley, Celestial Arts. (Kindle, 2013)**
I also love Dr Sara Buckley, a general practitioner and home birth activist. Her book provides lots of information about hormones and how they work during childbirth.

Calais-Germain, B. and Vives Pares, N. (2012). *Preparing for a Gentle Birth: The pelvis in pregnancy.* **Rochester: Healing Arts Press.**
A great book focusing on the anatomy of birth.

Dick-Read, G. (2004, sixth edition). *Childbirth Without Fear: The principles and practice of natural childbirth.* **London: Pinter & Martin.**
A classic to help you let go of your fears. Grantly Dick-Read's deep understanding of the nature of birth dates back over 60 years!

Gaskin, I. M. (2011). *A Midwife's Manifesto.* **London: Pinter & Martin.**
Any books written by Ina May Gaskin are wonderful. She really is my midwife hero and has been since I started out as a young midwife thirty years ago. She describes her experience and her amazing insights into natural birth so well, it's no surprise that she is world-famous and much in demand as a speaker. I love the birth talks that this spiritual midwife gives.

Gendlin, E. T. (2003). *Focusing: How to gain direct knowledge of your body's knowledge: How to open up your deeper feelings and intuitions.* **London: Rider.**

Gurmukh (2003). *Bountiful, Beautiful, Blissful: Experience the Natural Power of Pregnancy and Birth with Kundalini Yoga and Meditation*. New York: St Martin's Press. (Kindle edition available)
A great prenatal yoga book by a very famous Kundalini yogini.

Kataria, M. (2013). *Inner Spirit of Laughter – Five Secrets from the Laughing Guru*. Bangalore: Dr Kataria School of Laughter.

Leboyer, F. (1997). *Loving Hands: The traditional art of baby massage*. New York: Newmarket Press.

Leboyer, F. (1988). *Birth Without Violence*. New York: Random House.
I love Frederick Leboyer's books and his approach to gentle and natural childbirth, and was much influenced by him when I studied midwifery. *Birth Without Violence* changed the perspective on birth and babies forever, helping bring natural childbirth back to Europe. As early as the 1970s he acknowledged the baby as a real person with feelings, and in the 1980s he popularised baby massage. Merci beaucoup, Dr Frederick Leboyer!

Manitsas, K. (2011). *The Yoga of Birth: Sacred wisdom for conception, birthing and beyond*. lulu.com.
Katie is a beautiful friend of mine, a mother of four, a yoga teacher, and much else besides. Her book covers many different topics, including how to balance a busy family, a business and spirituality.

Mongan, M. (2015). *Hypnobirthing: The Mongan Method Revised Edition: A natural approach to a safe, easier and more comfortable birthing*. Deerfield Beach: Health Communications Inc.
Marie Mongan writes beautifully about the experience of giving birth; she is a hypnotherapist who has made hypnosis in childbirth very popular

Uvnas-Moberg, U (2011). *The Oxytocin Factor: Tapping the hormone of calm, love and healing.* London: Pinter & Martin. **(Kindle edition available)**
Fascinating if you want to find out more about oxytocin and research related to it.

Weed, S. (2012). *Wise Woman Herbal for the Childbearing Year.* **New Leaf Distribution Company. (Kindle edition available.)**
This book is also a classic, containing great herbal recipes that I love, and I've been working with homeopathy and herbs since 1987!

These are just a few of the excellent books out there that will help you to feel positive about your upcoming birth. Each one will give you its own perspective on this miraculous natural process.

DVDs

My hottest tips – these will really make a difference.

Babies (2010). **Directed by Thomas Balmès, US.**
This follows four babies in different cultures from birth through to their first steps. It's great fun to watch and gets you thinking about how you will bring up your own child.

The Big Stretch (2010). **Directed by Alieta Belle and Jenny Blyth, Australia.**
I love the great insights this DVD gives you on what women feel helped them through their labour. The beautiful births make you cry because they are so stunning.

Birth Day (2003), **directed by Diana Paul and Frank Ferrel, featuring Naoli Vinaver Lopez, US.**
Features a beautiful water birth, and shows how birth can be a

family experience – charming and delightful, makes you want to give birth.

***Birth into Being: birth as we know it.* Directed by Elena Tonetti-Vladimirova.**
Unusual DVD about water births in the ocean. Empowers the mind to see what women are capable of.

***Birth Without Violence* (2008). Frederick Leboyer, USA.**
A great choice if you want to see the difference it can make to babies to be delivered with gentleness and respect.

***Inner Strength* (2003). Midwifery team, Nussdorf, Austria. (Available from Birth International)**
'There are few topics which apply to all people equally – regardless of culture, colour of the skin and origin.' I agree wholeheartedly.

***Le Premier Cri* (2007). Directed by Gilles de Maistre, France.**
An exceptional film about childbirth in different parts of the world and how culture has a big influence on our birthing. Just great!

***Microbirths* (2014), directed by Toni Harman and Alex Wakeford, UK.**
My newest favourite: it talks about how bacteria and micro-organisms rule our health and our lives. It shows how important the correct balance of micro-organisms is, why we need to take care of our bacteria and the consequences this has for C-sections. An absolutely mind-blowing 'must watch'!

***What Babies Want* (2004). Directed by Debbie Takikawa, starring Noah Wyle, US.**
It opens a new universe, exploring how babies learn and develop in the womb.

Acknowledgements

So much time has passed since women first asked me to write this book. Thank you to all those women and babies, a spiral of infinity, who showed me the way. Thank you to all the wonderful people who encouraged me to sit down and set out my approach. Thanks to my lovely sister Usch, who gave me masses of support by just listening to me. Grazie to my extended family for the conversation at the family party that convinced me to write the book.

Cheers to Verity, who helped me find the right words in English, and an especial hooray for KPI and for Lucy, who taught me how to write a book and publish it.

Thanks to Betty my web designer and friend and all the beautiful friends and family that encouraged me to keep on going.

And of course I also give huge thanks to Elin Doka, who did the beautiful illustrations.

I am grateful to all the people I've met, friends and clients, who fill my life with their stories. You will find those stories and the learning from them in this book.

Thank you, too, to my beautiful teachers, who supported me and the birth of this book in their own ways. A book is like a seed that you carry around inside you, and then one day it wants to burst out and become a beautiful tree. Life itself, and everything and everyone in it, is a teacher that I bow my head to in thanks.

I know this is only a beginning, a step in the right direction, but I want to shout out a big thank you, *Dankeschön, grazie, gracias, merci, arigato, eyvallah, danevat* and above all... Happy Birth Day!

Praise for Jutta's methods

"Jutta has a wealth of knowledge and experience when it comes to birth and babies and I couldn't recommend her more highly for both her hypnobirthing sessions and her birthing classes. She's an incredibly calming influence – just what is needed when you're having a baby. We always looked forward to our time with Jutta and our only regret is that we didn't get in touch with her earlier, so we could have spent more time with her before the birth of our baby."

Rosina Budhani

The relationship a woman develops with her midwife is very special. From reading Jutta's website I liked the sound of her natural approach, and once I met her, I knew she was the midwife for me. My partner and I attended a birth preparation class with Jutta. The practical advice she gave us about breathing and massage techniques, different positions and so forth, made me feel prepared and excited rather than scared when I actually went into labour, and helped me immensely."

Lorraine

"During my pregnancy we went to see Jutta regularly, for a birthing preparation course, yoga classes and acupuncture. She taught us to have faith in the natural process of birthing and that the body and baby know just what to do. During the course and yoga classes, Jutta was able to support this with practical techniques that proved to be very helpful during labour. Thanks to these relaxation techniques, the labour turned out to be a very positive experience."

Charlotte and Vincent Heesbeen

"We found Jutta's preparation course for being parents very helpful for providing a positive perspective on birth. She shared her thirty years of experience as a midwife with us and explained how different techniques and different birth positions could enhance and support the natural birth process.

She also gave us a lot of advice on how we should communicate with the hospital about having a natural birth, and how we should avoid unnecessary medical intervention during the birth process and the negative consequences of this for mother and baby. We think this is vital information that new parents should definitely know before choosing a hospital. Finally, I had a quite smooth and natural birth, which I was so glad about and I felt so grateful for Jutta's knowledge."

We had a great experience with Jutta and her elements of birth. Many thanks to her, and I hope more women can enjoy the natural birth process for bringing their baby into the world.
Xiaoli

"Besides having over thirty years of experience and a vast amount of knowledge, Jutta also became a person I could go to express all my concerns and to receive reassurance. She helped me with pelvic pain by showing me great exercises to do as well as acupuncture. I also did a birthing class with her. After attending this class, my once sceptical husband decided to be there with me during the birth of our child. And I must say that thanks to all her advice he was the best coach I could have ever asked for. She is exactly what every mother-to-be needs. Without a doubt I would recommend her to every mother-to-be. Thank you, Jutta, for being so amazing!"
Kiran

"Your class addressed practical aspects of birthing, particularly the physiology of birth and the importance of the breath. You reminded us that birth is about surrendering to the mother's body – and the baby – and to 'not think', but rather, relax the face and body, and breathe. The class also provided helpful insights into the philosophy of birthing at a birth centre, reinforcing my sense that we had made the right choice in where to birth our baby."
Siobhan Toohill

"Being able to understand what I could do to help my partner while she was in the process of labour was very important to me. Before long we were all grimacing like Maori warriors (experimenting with a range of breathing techniques), having a laugh and learning how to let go at the same time. The best bit for me was the hypnosis at the end. To be reassured by the voice of experience is invaluable. For me it was the combination of Jutta's real-world knowledge and obvious spirituality that I found most generous and ultimately rewarding."
Peter and Maike

"The moment I walked into the Birthing Centre so distressed that I could go no further, Jutta's first words to me were, 'Breathe in' and I was hypnotised by her. Suddenly all my fears were gone and I knew that it would happen. No thoughts came into my mind except those that Jutta so positively gave me. At no point did I think of any pain killers. Jutta's words were intoxicating enough."
Vanessa and Franco Bortolin

"As two experienced doctors, we had not expected to learn so many interesting things about birth, given our medical backgrounds. I definitely recommend this childbirth course to all parents who want to learn about and understand the miracle of

birth, and want to be as well-prepared as they can. We travelled all the way from Cologne to Berlin to see and experience Jutta in person, and it was 100 per cent worth it."
Maria and Otto Iliadou

"I had a great birth. Without Jutta, I don't think I could have said that. It's as simple as that. She draws on so much experience and so many disciplines. But above all, it's her warmth and energy. She really cares and takes care of you. The Elements of Birth site was also such a fund of knowledge. I couldn't go to her antenatal course, but the online classes are something you can always go back to. I learnt so much more about how birth works – how crucial it is to prepare your mind (not just your body), and the incredible power of song and making noises!"
Abby Darcy

"We were very impressed by Jutta's openness to new insights (the results of research) while at the same time maintaining her commitment to established customs, and by the tireless effort she puts in when it comes to giving birth naturally.

Jutta gave us, both as a couple and individually, self-assurance and strength, so we knew we were on the right path. She empowered me to have trust in myself and my body, and to have faith in the force and the wisdom of Mother Nature."
Martin and Flavia

The Author

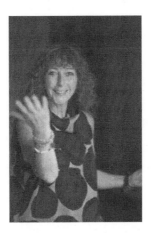

Teachers open the door but you must enter yourself

Jutta Wohlrab, midwife, entrepreneur, trainer, international speaker and founder of the Elements of Birth was born in Germany.

She trained to became a professional midwife in 1986 and has been passionate about supporting women, their partners and other birth professionals in how to achieve the best pregnancy and birth ever since.

Jutta has trained in homeopathy for midwives, acupuncture for midwives, hypnosis and hypnotherapy, is a trained yoga teacher and trainer, and NLP Trainer. She has lived and practised in three different countries and gained much knowledge working in different birthing environments.

Jutta loves to inspire people through all aspects of her work. She truly believes in times of so much intervention and fear around childbirth it is time to bring back the happiness and joy.

She likes to share the best of everything, not only in her workshops and trainings but also at conferences and in her online programme.

Jutta has had articles published and featured on the radio in the UK, Canada and Australia. She lives in Berlin and Australia and as a people person enjoys sharing her knowledge around all aspects of pregnacy, birth and the time after all around the world.

Happy Birthing Days is not just a book, it is also an online program that I have created. I had great fun filming all the video tutorials for the program and the feedback from mothers and their birthing partners around the world has been overwhelmingly positive. I love to help as many people as possible and if you are reading this book then you can get 20% off the online program and any off my other programs; it is my way of saying thank you.

All you have to do is go to my website, www.elementsofbirth.com and use the coupon code HBDBOOK20.

Printed in Great Britain
by Amazon